from burnout to balance

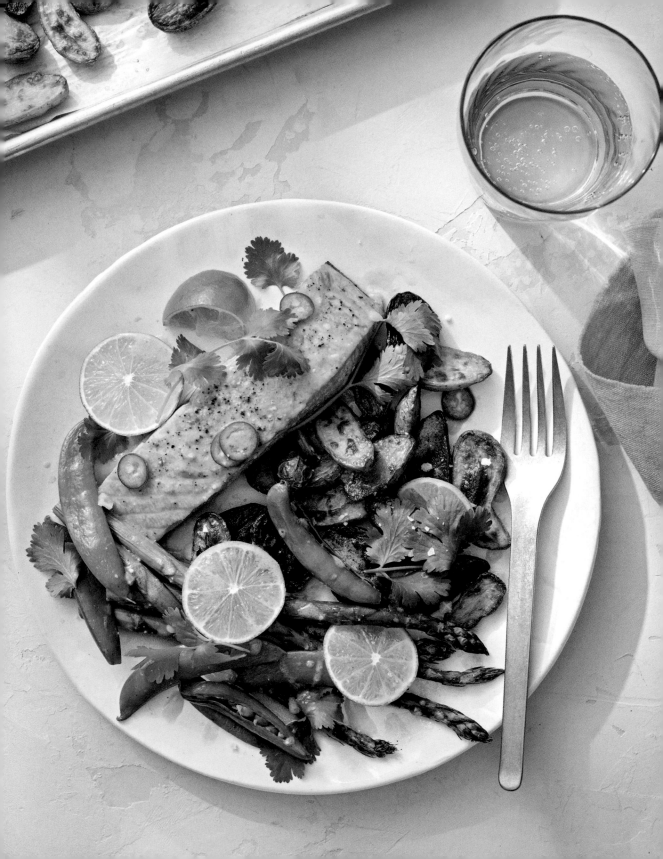

from burnout to balance

60+ healing recipes & simple strategies to boost mood, immunity, focus, & sleep

PATRICIA BANNAN, MS, RDN

Fountaindale Public Library District
300 W. Briarcliff Rd.
Bolingbrook, IL 60440

RODALE
BOOKS

Copyright © 2022 by Patricia Bannan
All rights reserved.

Published in the United States by Rodale Books,
an imprint of Random House, a division of Penguin
Random House LLC, New York.

rodalebooks.com

RODALE and the Plant colophon are registered
trademarks of Penguin Random House LLC.

Library of Congress Cataloging-in-Publication Data
is available upon request.

ISBN 978-0-593-23242-2
eBook ISBN 978-0-593-23243-9

Printed in China

Food Stylist: Haley Hazell
Prop Stylist: Nidia Cueva
Photographer: Jennifer Chong

Editor: Donna Loffredo
Designer: Jan Derevjanik
Production Editor: Serena Wang
Production Manager: Heather Williamson
Composition: Merri Ann Morrell and Zoe Tokushige
Copy Editor: Laura Cherkas
Indexer: Jay Kreider

10 9 8 7 6 5 4 3 2 1

First Edition

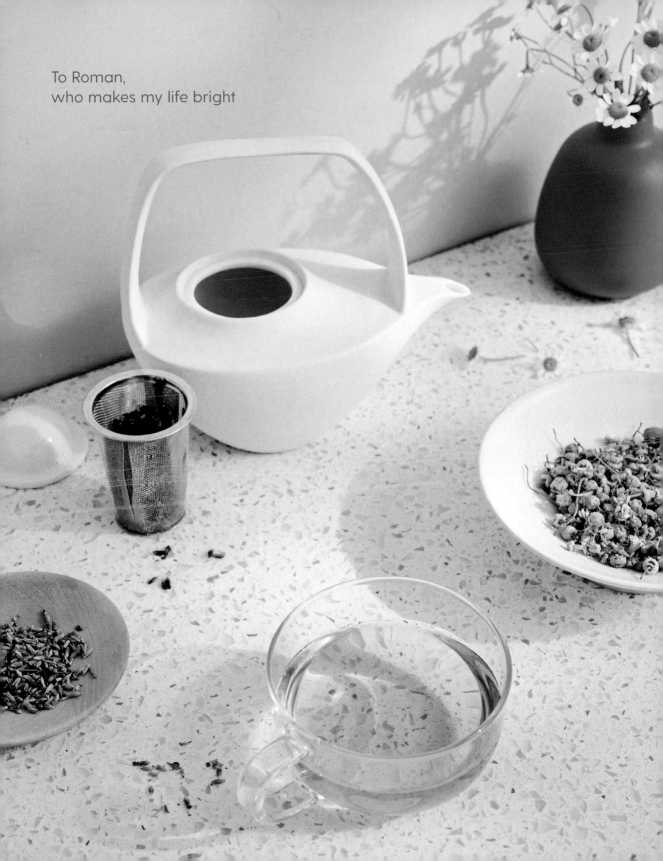

To Roman,
who makes my life bright

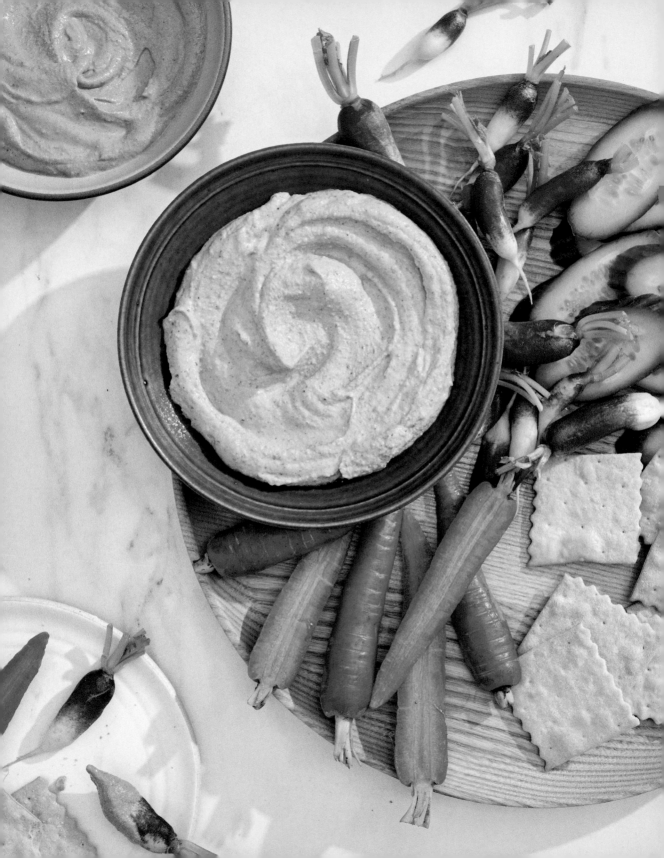

contents

female burnout

when your double-espresso vodka latte just doesn't cut it anymore

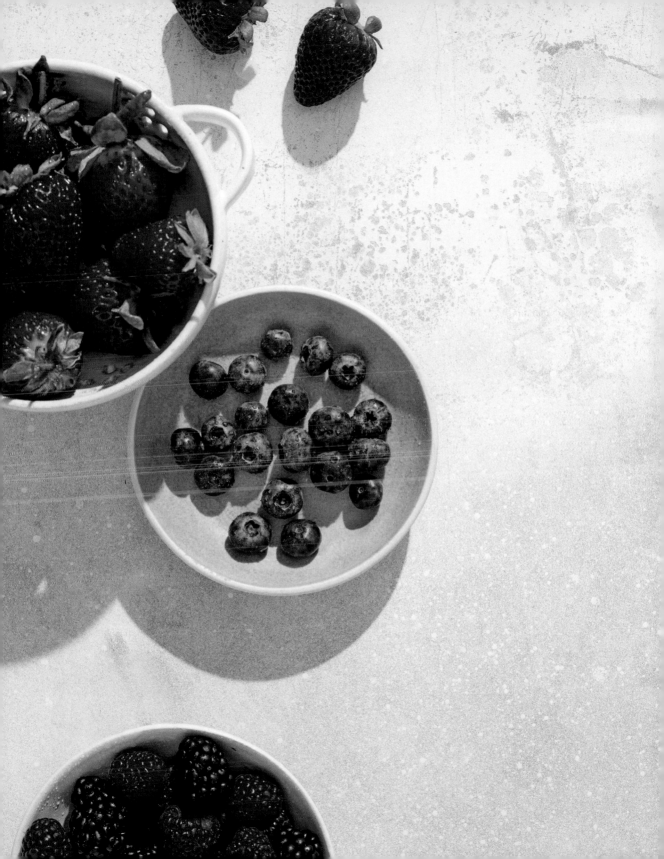

> I walk around like everything is fine,
> but deep down, inside my shoe,
> my sock is sliding off.
> —Anonymous

We've all had those days. On the outside, we seem like we have it all together. But on the inside, it's a different story. Sure, it's just a loose sock, but it's annoying—and it's throwing off your gait more with every step. But you can't stop or slow down, so you tell yourself that you can smile through it. That it's not noticeable. That you're fine, it's fine, *everything's fine.*

Then, thanks to the "pretending everything is fine" game you're playing (and the sock that is now balled up somewhere under your arch), you stumble and turn your ankle. Well done! Now it actually hurts when you walk. *Could it be broken? You do not have time for a broken ankle.*

So you power through. You sit down for the rest of the day, slyly ice your throbbing ankle under your desk, and hobble to your car as you joke to your colleagues that it's nothing. You've got this!

Yes, you've "got" this. But what do you have? A sprained ankle, a wounded ego, and a bad habit of ignoring tiny problems that snowball into big ones? And what is the cost?

I'll tell you what the cost was for me: nearly everything I had worked so hard to build personally and professionally. Does that sound a little dramatic? Yeah, it does, but it's true. I was so burned out, dried up, hollowed out, sucked dry that I was a fire hazard. Light a match near me and stand back. Stick a fork in me. I'm done.

In my early forties, I hit a wall. I "had it all," after years of personal challenges that included financial dips, career shifts, falling in love with a man with a child and eventually marrying him, embracing a blended family, and, most stressful of all, trying to get pregnant through IVF.

I was worn-out to my limits (and beyond) for years. But finally, after countless sleepless nights and nail-biting days, I had a terrific husband, a wonderful stepson, and the most beautiful, healthy daughter I could have imagined.

Instead of feeling elated, however, I found myself lying on a massage table six months after my baby was born, completely and utterly depleted. I was there to relax, but instead I felt empty, exhausted, and worn. I loved my family so much, but at that time, caring for them made me feel like I had nothing left for myself. And, frankly, I didn't feel like I was doing my best job caring for them, either.

It was like the day after pulling an all-nighter for an exam, when you finally allow your body and your brain to crash. But my "all-nighter" had lasted half a decade! My tank was past *E* and I was running on fumes. I couldn't relax. I couldn't cry. I couldn't worry. I just couldn't. (That phrase "can't even"? Yeah, that was me.)

At first, I didn't know what was wrong. I wasn't depressed. I wasn't stressed anymore. I wasn't angry. I only felt empty. Scorched. Crispy, like a leaf that dries out and curls up in the midday sun. My vibrant essence and drive—and my type A personality, which had carried me through college and grad school, through my constantly on-the-go twenties and thirties—all that was gone. This wasn't aging or your run-of-the-mill postpartum exhaustion. It was something different.

What I later learned was that I was experiencing burnout. I had spent so long in fight-or-flight mode, forcing my adrenal glands to work overtime, that I had no energy left. Right there, on that massage table, I started to understand what was going on. My body did, too. It realized things were finally (finally!) okay, so it could just shut down. The problem was—I couldn't get it started again.

I quickly realized this wasn't a situation that a massage or a martini with my girlfriends could fix. Even a spa weekend couldn't begin to touch it. I needed a few months of R&R—not the cushy, woo-woo, self-care version, but the real, deep, restorative type.

I needed to get back to basics. I needed regular sleep—not a double latte and better concealer. I needed to eat real, simple food—not protein bars or green juices while running between appointments. And I needed to move my body—not to lose weight or sculpt my arms but to feel healthy and deal with stress. Mostly, I needed to listen to myself again. I needed to tune in to the voice inside my head that had warned me I was pushing too hard.

Even though I'm a registered dietitian with more than two decades of experience and a graduate degree, I had lost sight of the things that matter most when it comes to health. But I also knew (and I experienced firsthand as I reconnected with them) that these "basics" were going to bring me back to *me*.

So I sat down with my husband, told him what was going on, and explained that I needed to take a step back from work and other obligations to make time for my health and myself. We took a temporary financial hit. It was hard, but it had to happen.

I focused on breathing (I know, it sounds silly, but it works), exercise, food, and sleep. I did all the things I had been telling my clients to do but wasn't making time to do myself. And you know what? It worked. Not only that, but when I started to emerge from this zombielike state and share my story with my colleagues, girlfriends, and the other moms at drop-off, so many of them could relate. They too had burned out and dried up. Over and over, I heard their stories:

- The tech sales executive who ignored her stress for so long that she ended up having to go on short-term disability to heal her physical and mental health

- The optician who went on autopilot when her husband was diagnosed with a benign brain tumor that manifested as "sudden-onset dementia" in his early forties

- The recruiter who started to notice that nothing else provided the same release as a couple of glasses of wine—and wondered if that was the start of a bigger problem

- The colleague who was sick more often than not despite living in Los Angeles, working out regularly, and "drinking more green juice than ever"

All these women have different jobs, live in different cities, and have different home situations. But our stories overlap. We ignored ourselves to tune in to what everyone else in our lives needed. And we nearly ended up a smoldering pile of ashes in the process.

That's when I knew I had to write this book. For myself, for those women, and for women like you who deserve to feel whole again. Throughout this book, you'll meet some of those women as they share their stories in their own words.

You can have it all— but what's the price?

You can have it all, my generation of women heard over and over. But they left out the important part: *Just not all at once.* We start stretching ourselves thin earlier than you might realize. At school, we study around the clock while navigating social circles and keeping up with the extracurriculars that help us stand out. In our twenties, we throw ourselves into climbing the career ladder— while learning to be adults and searching for our soul mates! Then, as mothers we are expected to work like we don't have children to raise while raising children like we don't work outside the home. It never ends.

I love being a mom and a stepmom. I love being a wife. And I love my work. But I, like most women, could really use another, oh, thirty-six hours in a day—and maybe a clone who can help with the laundry and the dishes. My cost for trying to "have it all" was burnout. And I'm not alone. We're paying the price for buying into the idea that we have to push through, bear the burden alone, and excel in every area of our lives at the time same.

The cost for most women and the cost for society

Burnout affects women differently than it does men (more on that later) and it affects us more often. In 2019, Meredith Corp and the Harris Poll teamed up to get a feel on the level of stress women are facing today. Compared with five years prior, women said they felt stressed, tired, anxious, overwhelmed—you get the picture—at significantly higher levels than the men surveyed.

Women were more likely than men to struggle with:

- Sleeping
- Concentration
- Completing chores
- Maintaining healthy eating habits
- Decisions or planning for the future

Half of the women said they felt they were just going through the motions every day, but at the same time, over three-quarters said they put their family's needs ahead of their own, 60 percent said they didn't get enough "me time," and 60 percent said that when they skimped on their own self-care, they were less productive.

Two-thirds of women said they felt like they worked a full day before leaving for the office in the morning. The "sandwich generation"—comprising 30 million women who are simultaneously caring for an older parent while raising their own children—feels this most profoundly (73 percent).

We're also better than men at hiding burnout: According to the 2017 State of the American Workplace Report from Gallup, women are more engaged than their male counterparts at work—and they have been for as long as the analytics firm has been tracking that measurement.

The price of having it all

Burnout feels like a decidedly modern problem, but burning the candle at both ends has happened since long before we earned the right to vote. Before burnout had the official "endorsement" of the World Health Organization, we had all sorts of euphemisms for it: exhaustion, hysteria, the vapors . . . Whatever we call it, now we know it's not "all in our heads."

It's in our lives. Our always-too-busy, always-on-the-go, always-one-step-behind, trying-to-squeeze-in-just-one-more-thing lives.

The poet Edna St. Vincent Millay warned us back in 1918:

> My candle burns at both ends;
> It will not last the night;
> But ah, my foes, and oh, my friends—
> It gives a lovely light!

A candle burning at both ends is a fire hazard, friends. Getting too close is a recipe for disaster. It's burned skin and singed hair and blaring fire alarms just waiting to happen. Sounds a lot like your mood during burnout, doesn't it?

After 9/11, we saw an uptick in compassion fatigue and burnout among the "helpers"—first responders, social workers, and clergy.

We also saw an increase in PTSD among those who were seriously impacted. Natural disasters like the deadly wildfires in California, where I live, or hurricanes such as Katrina or Rita, can lead to the same.

And I know in my heart we'll see something similar in the coming years now that we've lived through the COVID-19 pandemic. During the stressful and scary time of sheltering in place, I read story after story of women being pushed to their limits—little to no child care support, working from home, struggling with lost work, extra emotional labor, not to mention the fear and anxiety that go along with so much uncertainty and stress.

A couple of months into staying "safe at home," I read a piece by Arianna Huffington, whose own burnout led to her literal collapse back in 2007. She calls COVID-19 a crucible that "revealed fundamental weaknesses in our society—many of which we knew about but were content to ignore." Huffington suggests we view the pandemic as an opportunity to change, a chance to rise from the ashes and bring with us only what works—and leave behind or replace everything else.

You get that same opportunity as you heal and move forward from burnout. For Mireille, that meant plotting to leave her eighty-hour-a-week job and move home to Europe. It meant putting an hourlong walk on her calendar every single day without fail.

For Tamika, it meant giving up a high-powered position where she collected achievements, praise, and bonuses like brass rings. Instead, she learned to be okay with "not being the best." She's still providing for her family and living a comfortable life, only now it's a life where she gets to be present.

Why doesn't everyone burn out?

In talking to other women, I found that each one felt alone—like she was the only one who couldn't hack it as a supermom, star employee, beloved wife, and best friend. One interesting perspective on stress comes from Dr. Leanne Williams, founder of Stanford University's Center for Precision Mental Health and Wellness. With her team, she identified specific subtypes for depression and anxiety.

These "biotypes" are:

- Rumination (worrying repeatedly and getting "stuck" in negative thought cycles)

- Anxious avoidance (avoiding situations that cause stress)

- Threat dysregulation (staying in fight-or-flight mode after a threat has passed)

- Anhedonia (losing interest in pleasurable activities or experiences)

- Cognitive dyscontrol (inability to control emotions, behaviors, thoughts, etc.)

- Inattention (struggling to concentrate and focus)

During the pandemic, Dr. Williams shared that our biotype—which can be observed in part via MRI—impacts not only depression and anxiety but also how we adapt to stress. And once we know how we adapt to stress, we start to notice when we're experiencing it—so we can avoid letting it progress toward burnout!

Is this burnout—or just stress?

By now you might be wondering about the difference between burnout and stress. While chronic, unrelenting stress can lead to burnout, the symptoms are different. That's because burnout is stress that's taken such a toll that you no longer feel like yourself. While stress—even intense bouts of it—might motivate you to work harder and parent "better," burnout makes you feel like you can't function and no longer want to.

Stress can and will take a toll on your physical and emotional health. Think of it like going into debt because you keep putting everything on credit cards.

Stress happened when Rebecca watched the medical bills pile up after her husband's brain surgery, when her boss threatened to fire her for missing work to care for him, and when she stepped into her husband's role as the breadwinner, the protector, and the one who took care of everyone.

Burnout is when you've maxed out those cards, drained your savings, maybe bounced some checks, and don't have even a dime left to your name.

Burnout happened when Rebecca was so stressed out that she stopped caring—when she told her boss to go ahead and fire her, when she would get into bed at night and realize her whole day had been spent on autopilot, and when she was "no longer living—only functioning and doing one thing at a time to 'just keep going.'"

HERE'S A COMPARISON:

Stress	Burnout
I have a full to-do list. I feel overly involved with or connected to every task.	I feel disconnected from work and home. I don't care about any of it. I feel like I'm going through the motions.
I have a short fuse or cry at the drop of a hat. I can't *not* react.	I don't really react emotionally anymore. I'm unfazed.
I'm tired. I have no energy.	I feel hopeless. I have no energy.
I feel overwhelmed.	I feel empty or numb.
I can feel this affecting me physically.	I'm feeling mostly emotional side effects.

How stressed are you?

Burnout doesn't happen in a vacuum, and you don't "catch" it randomly, like the common cold. Stress builds faster than you can deal with it, and eventually you're so buried by it that your body gives up and burns out.

Women are especially good at bearing heavy loads and thinking *I'm fine* or *It's not that bad* or *My friend/neighbor/sister has it much harder than I do.*

How burned out are you?

Burnout was first measured on the Maslach Burnout Inventory, which divides burnout into three different dimensions:

1. **Emotional exhaustion:** You feel stuck, trapped, like you have no control over your life due to chronic stress that has eroded your resilience.

   Mireille thought her burnout was just fatigue from caring for two kids, commuting between the suburbs and New York City, and learning to navigate life and work in a new country.

2. **Depersonalization:** You start to become detached from yourself and your life. You don't care about things that used to bring you joy, and you feel less connection to people (even your kids or sweetheart) and your work.

   Lisa saw this manifest as constant activity solely for the sake of distraction. Travel, partying, workouts, and working late filled her days, but she didn't enjoy any of it. "I was mentally drained, but I was just trying to avoid my thoughts, so I ran myself ragged," she says.

3. **Lack of accomplishment:** You take less pride in your work (both at home and at the office), and you begin to doubt that you know what you're doing. You start doing less or scaling back, but not in a strategic way that will heal burnout.

   For Jacqueline, a successful photographer, this led to doubt in her talents, wondering what her purpose was in life, and questioning whether she should quit all she had built for herself.

While this burnout self-test was developed for occupational burnout, you can't ignore that it happens in our personal lives, too. As a practitioner, I think it's important we realize the holistic nature and enmeshed causes of burnout. I often discuss the three pillars of burnout as: work stress, personal challenges, and personality type. If you're like me, a type A perfectionist or people-pleaser, you're likely more prone to burnout than your laid-back friend.

Are you burning out?

Not sure whether you've experienced burnout (or are experiencing it right now)? Here's a quick checklist of common symptoms:

- Anxiety and/or depression
- Changes in productivity and work or home performance
- Constantly feeling tired or fatigued, for no known reason
- Feeling apathetic, hopeless, or defenseless
- Feeling more negative than usual or isolated
- Getting sick more often than usual
- Irritability and feeling raw
- Loss of appetite or eating more sugary or carb-filled foods than usual
- No longer enjoying things you once did
- Physical symptoms like headaches, shortness of breath, chest tightness, stomach upset
- Rage and anger
- Shorter attention span and difficulty concentrating
- Trouble sleeping due to a racing mind, waking up throughout the night, or insomnia

How many of these describe how you're feeling? If you have more than a few, you might be experiencing burnout.

Ready for a silver lining? Burnout doesn't have to be permanent—neither does depression or anxiety. And researchers have found that there's often a rebound effect. After experiencing our lowest lows, we feel *higher* highs.

Those times when you're cranky and can't pull yourself out of it are a coping mechanism. When you're not happy, your brain shifts strategies to better deal with the hard stuff—and you become more empathetic, too.

A deal with the devil: How you pay for burnout eventually

Don't fall prey to the idea that burnout is simply the price women pay for having it all—or that it's all in your head. Nope. Burnout has real, physical consequences for your health and well-being, including:

Your heart

In 2020, a study published in the *European Journal of Preventive Cardiology* reported a connection between severe burnout (aka vital exhaustion) and a type of irregular heartbeat called atrial fibrillation.

Burnout may also be a risk factor for coronary heart disease, a condition that about eight in ten women ages forty to sixty are at risk of developing.

Further, a study by the American Friends of Tel Aviv University discovered that scoring high on a burnout scale (in the top 20 percent) led to a 79 percent increase in risk of coronary disease for healthy men and women!

Weight gain

This is one side effect of burnout that likely doesn't need a study to back it up—but one exists! Researchers confirmed, in a study published in 2019 in the *Journal of Health Psychology,* that it is harder to keep up with healthy habits when you're exhausted, which can lead to weight gain.

Plus, when we're stressed, our bodies store calories differently, because our cortisol levels are higher. Our hormones are hardwired in a way that could lead to weight gain when we're stressed—or burned—out.

Diabetes and metabolic syndrome

Stress is a potential cause for type 2 diabetes and metabolic syndrome, a group of conditions that raises your risk for heart disease, diabetes, and stroke, among other things.

A 2006 study looked at the connection between work stress and metabolic syndrome. While more men were at risk, they were only twice as likely to have metabolic syndrome; in women, the group was smaller, but the likelihood was higher (over five times!).

Autoimmune conditions

While the research is still new—and certainly stress isn't the only cause—autoimmune conditions have been linked to stress-related disorders, including PTSD. Chronic stress, which turns into burnout, can lead to chronic inflammation—the root cause of so many diseases and conditions.

And on top of all that, there's what burnout does to your brain . . .

This is your brain on burnout

Think back to that PSA from the 1980s where a fried egg in a pan is supposed to be "your brain on drugs." Something similar happens when you're burned out—your brain physically changes, and not in a good way.

- **Your amygdala gets bigger.** That's the part of the brain in charge of your emotional responses. If you feel like you're jumpier than usual and too quick to react, that's why.

- **Your prefrontal cortex thins.** That's the area of the brain that handles cognitive function. If you're struggling to juggle work and home schedules like you used to, blame that change in your brain.

- **Your memory and attention are impacted**—and your brain begins to physically resemble the brain of someone who's suffered severe emotional trauma.

- **Your connections and synapses dull,** making it harder to be creative, stay focused, and turn out quality work the way you once did.

By now you might be wondering: Why is this happening? There are so many contributing factors—keeping up with others around you, trying to be everything to everyone all the time, feeling like you aren't able to share how you really feel, feeling isolated despite your constant online connection—but they all come down to this:

Our lives are a lot harder than our bodies are designed to handle.

Why stress happens

Stress is as natural to your body as digestion or breathing—we're hardwired to experience it so we can stay safe in the face of danger. Ideally, we feel occasional bursts of stress from real or imagined threats, and that sets off our body's fight-or-flight response, via our sympathetic nervous system.

Back in ancient times, this saved lives: when the saber-toothed tiger came to the village, your ancestor was ready to run, her babies tucked safely under her arms. Today, you draw on this same instinct when you need to quickly stop your child from running into the street or slam on the brakes to avoid an accident.

In your body, your adrenals—two almond-shaped glands that rest on your kidneys toward the back of your body—are in charge of keeping stress in check. They do this by regulating the release of hormones like cortisol and adrenaline, and they also use cortisol to manage your sleep-wake cycle. When your cortisol levels are normal and in balance, you're a more resilient, happier, healthier person.

Your adrenals have help from your hypothalamus and pituitary gland. This trio is known as the HPA axis, and together they assess and deal with all of life's challenges.

Your body is a well-oiled machine that can adapt and handle a lot, but it also *really* just likes to stay steady and balanced, in a state of equilibrium. When it comes to stress, it prefers this scenario:

1. Danger happens. Your body reacts: you go into fight-or-flight mode.

2. You get to safety, and your body returns to rest-and-digest mode.

3. Your body stays there until the next stressor appears—maybe next week or next month.

But *equilibrium* and *balance* aren't exactly words most of us would associate with our lives. We have far more than that "normal, occasional" stress. So what happens? We get stuck in "on" mode, and we're constantly reacting like we're in danger—even when we're safe in our beds, trying to get some sleep.

The longer stress goes on, the harder it is to find balance—and the more areas of your body are affected. You're not sleeping well, so you're not eating right, and you're getting sick all the time. Your stomach hurts—that was my sign. Chronic stress can impact every single area of your body and your mind.

You can find that balance again, though, and you can build resilience, which is your body's secret weapon for taking on every challenge that comes your way. You'll learn how to rebuild that resilience and heal yourself, one day—and one meal—at a time.

The generation gap and burnout

I first started researching women and burn-out after I'd found my way out of it and while I was hearing stories from my Generation X peers. Back then, I assumed I knew which subsets of women were the most stressed: women around my age, going through the same things I was. I thought that many millennials were still too young to be burned out—that younger millennials in their 20s are still relatively early in their careers, and they may not be parents or homeowners yet. I share all this as a preface to the shock of discovering that millennials (adults born between the years 1981 and 1996) are the burnout generation.

Millennials are dealing with the same work demands and stagnant wages as other generations, and they're feeling the burden of not having a financial cushion or many wins under their belt at this stage of life. They're earning less than their boomer parents, and some headlines go as far as saying they're seeing the "American Dream collapsing" for their generation. According to a report on the Blue Cross Blue Shield Health Index, their mental health is suffering, with a 47 percent rise in diagnoses of major depression since 2013 for their age group.

Partly due to the financial stress of student-loan debt, health care, child care, and an expensive housing market, more of them are dying young, according to the public health groups Trust for America's Health and Well Being Trust. These heartbreaking "deaths of despair" are related to alcohol, drugs, and suicide, and we lost 36,000 millennials this way in 2017 alone. And while we hear more about loneliness among older adults, it's millennials who lack social support and are feeling the effects of isolation mentally and physically.

Burnout is also related to demographics and life experience—and Black and Indigenous women, and women of color face additional hurdles and systemic inequities that can exacerbate their stress and interfere with their ability to get help. In fact, many demographics of women are more impacted by burnout in markedly different ways, such as single moms, those living at or below the poverty line, those who identify as LGBTQ+, and women who feel unsafe in their homes.

I share all this to say: no matter where you are in life, you can burn out—but you can also reignite your inner spark. This book is for you.

So what can you do about burnout?

If you're burned out, there's hope. You don't have to feel like this forever, and you can start to feel more like yourself as soon as today. From learning the importance of saying no, to practically zero-effort meals and snacks, to simplifying your decision-making process, this book is packed with science-based strategies, meal plans, and more than sixty delicious recipes to help you reclaim your life. Food is such a crucial component for dealing with burnout. As a dietitian, I've seen the healing power of food with my clients, and I've seen it in my own life. I'm here to help you do the same, so you can feel your best. Plus, I offer lifestyle tools to help you beyond the kitchen, since burnout impacts all parts of you.

In the next chapter you will learn how to adopt a "back to basics" food and lifestyle plan to beat burnout. You'll learn how to simplify your life, starting in the kitchen, with an overview of what to eat to beat burnout, time- and budget-saving food strategies, and a one-week meal plan.

The following chapters provide more specific nutrition and lifestyle information to help you target the area where you struggle most. I know you have limited time and energy, so start with the food overview in chapter 2, then skip to the chapter that most strongly applies to your life. The four core symptoms of burnout addressed in this book are mood (chapter 3), immunity (chapter 4), focus (chapter 5), and sleep (chapter 6). After that, move on to the other chapters as you're able.

Each of these topic chapters offers a top twenty-five food list so you can quickly start eating foods that help you overcome your biggest challenge, whether that's a better mood, fewer sick days, enhanced focus, or a good night's sleep. A one-week meal plan is also provided in each of these chapters that specifically targets what you need most.

In chapter 7 you will find a collection of sixty-plus delicious plant-centric recipes to help you beat burnout. Many of these recipes are included in the meal plans as well.

Let's get started.

chapter 2

burnout busters

taking care of yourself when it feels too overwhelming

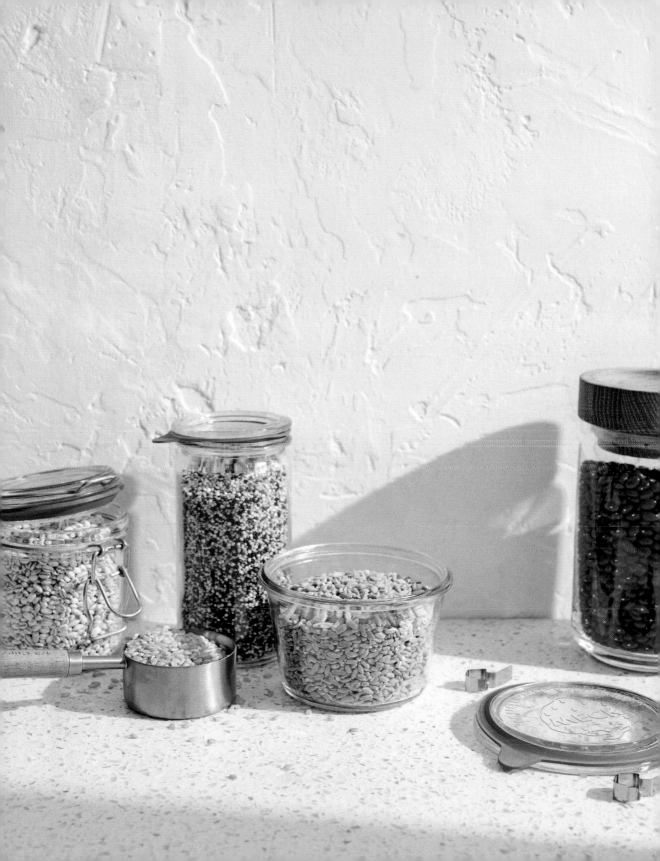

> Almost everything will work again if you unplug
> it for a few minutes . . . including you.
> —Anne Lamott

When you've grown accustomed to living in a certain way—even if that way involves heaps of stress, anguish, and exhaustion—change seems daunting, and even more tiring. But now that you've learned about what burnout is doing to your health and your life, there's no turning back.

Change doesn't happen overnight, and your body is going to need more than a few minutes of unplugging to regain its balance. (But anytime you can unplug for a few minutes, do it—those minutes will add up.) Whether you're talking about weight loss, training for a marathon, or undoing years of accumulated stress and exhaustion, small steps lead to big changes. You will make progress. You might also hit a plateau—or even "relapse." But you can (and will) feel better. You don't have to live in burnout or teeter on the edge of it. You can find your way back to a calmer, happier, more fulfilled way of living.

I don't have a cure or miracle to offer you. But I can show you how to identify burnout triggers and symptoms, like I did. I can teach you what to do and how to respond when burnout creeps in, something that took me trial and error to figure out. And, of course, as a registered dietitian, I can teach you about the foods and nutrients that will help boost your mood, support your immunity, enhance

your focus, and improve your sleep—all things that will help you feel more like you again. I've created recipes that maximize the foods that can support you as you heal, all quick and easy to make (because the last thing you need is to add "become a gourmet chef" to your to-do list), which you'll find in chapter 7. And I can help you understand that the little voice inside your head is wiser than you know. As Glinda says to Dorothy at the end of *The Wizard of Oz:* "You had the power all along, my dear."

For me, one of the keys to getting out of burnout was saying no to friends and work opportunities more than I'd like (hello, FOMO trigger!). It meant letting go of the idea of buying my dream house in favor of living somewhere smaller and more financially and logistically manageable. And it meant making room for a lot of little habits that help me invest in myself and my healing. I certainly don't do these things perfectly, or all the time, but it helps when I try:

- Keeping my kitchen stocked with nourishing (and time-saving) essentials

- Turning my phone off at night to limit my time on social media

- Telling my husband what I'm grateful for when I find myself complaining

- Doing some physical activity *most* days (even if it's just a ten-minute yoga class online)

- Taking shortcuts where and how I can—without making myself feel guilty

- Learning where to cut corners and bend the rules so I don't break

This chapter serves two purposes: It provides helpful burnout "busters," tips and tricks that can buy you some time, help you save money, and conserve your energy. And it'll also help you get set up for success in the kitchen, since so much of this plan is about food. By the end of the chapter, you'll have a better idea of what you can do today to set yourself on the right path.

Delegate or Let It Go

You have to learn to delegate, says Jacqueline, and that's tough—especially when you're used to being in charge of it all. Most importantly, "You can't worry about what other people will think if you ask for help or take things off your plate."

She advises, "If there are things you can ask of others that you don't want to do, don't have the expertise to do, or don't have the time to do (as in you'll lose sleep or sanity if you do it), just let it go. Either let someone else do it or let no one do it. It's surprising how many things I've let go of that ultimately no one cares about. Once they were gone, I realized I didn't miss them, either."

Maybe you stop organizing monthly office outings or you let another parent figure out the end-of-season gifts for the coaches. What would happen if you brought store-bought cookies to the Halloween party instead of homemade? Or gave gift cards instead of personalized gifts?

Talk about a relief!

How to beat burnout:
Go back to basics and simplify your life

Here in America, we live in a "more, more, more" society where we're expected to keep up with the Joneses online and IRL. Meanwhile, we have no safety net and feel ourselves pulled in every direction.

So how do we simplify? How do we get back to basics?

This will look different for everyone. Only you know what really matters to you—and what weighs most heavily on you. Start by asking yourself a few questions and assessing how you currently divide your time.

- At the end of each day, if you look back over your day, where do you feel like you wasted the most time? What demanded more of your energy than it was worth?
  Examples: *packing lunches for all three kids, arguing with your son about picking out clothes, scrolling through social media, watching TV*

- What do you want to spend more time doing each day but can't, due to other obligations?
  Examples: *sleeping eight hours, working on your own projects, exercising*

- What is the biggest source of stress for you?
  Examples: *money, keeping the house clean, a job you dislike, parenting responsibilities, no time for yourself, all of the above*

- If money were no object, what type of help would you like to have?
  Examples: *a nanny or babysitter, a massage therapist on call, a personal chef, a housekeeper*

Let these answers guide you as you start to decide what to keep and what to shed.

How Real Women Win the Battle against Burnout

"I run, I do yoga, and I meditate. Those help me immensely. And I think about Banksy's words: 'If you get tired, learn to rest, not to quit.'" —Tamika

"I have to have healthy boundaries. I'm more likely to get sick, run down, and feel more tired if I don't. I go see a therapist and let it all out." —Pippa

"Accept help! I can't emphasize the support part enough—it means something different to all of us. But if you can get help, take it, even if it's not the help you want (say, from your ex or a neighbor you don't like much). It'll give you a chance to take a break from drinking from the firehose." —Maribel

"I found something besides wine. In retrospect, I drank a lot. I could see that that could become a problem. I release from a couple of glasses of wine—it really works. But that dependence wasn't something I wanted to keep." —Tamika

"Medication was a game-changer. I really fought it, and I called my therapist to tell them I didn't want to be on it. But I took it. A month later, I found my words again. I felt like myself. I regretted not doing it sooner. Shortly after, I left my job, too." —Lisa

"Yoga helped me work through a lot: postpartum depression, miscarriages, a big move, when my marriage was not in a good place, then my divorce. Through it all, yoga has really been amazing for me. It's my physical version of mental therapy (though I love that, too). I tell fellow divorced moms: you have to put your oxygen mask on first." —Kimball

"When I get in my own head, I talk to my people—I have a close circle. I go to my husband, my best friend, or my business partner. Getting their input helps." —Lisa

"Once you've dealt with depression or anxiety, any bad mood can be scary—you worry that you'll be in it for six months. After a couple of rough spots, I realized I could just say to myself, 'Hey, I just hit a bump in the road. I'll be okay.'" —Kimball

"When my husband got sick and I slipped into burnout, I focused on what I could control—a home improvement project, a task at work, or helping my son with his homework. I tried to tune out what I couldn't control." —Rebecca

"My friends and I send voice memos when we are too busy to talk. You have to find ways to make it work. Lower the bar if you need to but don't quit. When you're really 'in the shit,' it's hard, but you have to try." —Kimball

"Cognitive behavioral therapy gave me the steps to learn to cope. I started by getting rid of catastrophic thinking. I hold myself to a certain standard, and it's hard to see anything but 100 percent effort as success. But I am successful. I have a great marriage. I am a good parent. We need more empathy for ourselves." —Tamika

In case of emergency, break glass

These habits and practices won't fix the root cause of your burnout, but they can help you get through a rough day. Keep these in your back pocket the next time you need a quick fix to ease some stress or find the joy.

- **Check your breath.** When you feel your heart beating faster and the panic creeping in, pause and close your eyes. Listen to your breath—and place a hand on your heart if you're able. Take three deep breaths as you tune out everything else.

- **Find connection.** Send a text or a DM to a friend. Call your mom or brother. Pop over to your coworker's desk. When you feel like you're going it alone, prove yourself wrong by reminding yourself you have people.

- **Go outside.** Never underestimate the power of fresh air and/or sunshine. Even a few minutes in the parking lot instead of a windowless office can help you refresh. As you'll read in coming chapters, your immune system, mood, and sleep cycle will all thank you!

- **Make a list.** Not a to-do list but a gratitude list. Jot down a few things in your life (the big ones and the not-so-big ones) that make you feel thankful. Keep the list handy for next time. (My list might include dark chocolate, my backyard garden, and my kids, for example.)

- **Remind yourself "why."** Have a thesis deadline looming? Stressed out by all the laundry that comes with three little ones? Feeling pushed to the edge by your patients or clients? Remind yourself why you made these choices in the first place, as a way to carry you through the harder days.

- **Schedule self-care.** Start to block out time for yourself. It might be five minutes to meditate or an hour to run. It might be a solo evening out or a weekend when you can sleep in and leave parenting to your partner. If it's in your calendar, it's a commitment—so don't cancel. Sometimes knowing I have an hour set aside for myself on a Friday afternoon gets me through the week.

- **Unplug your phone.** Notifications can become distractions and intrusions when you're overwhelmed. Turn them off for a while so you can focus. Set your phone to airplane mode to buy yourself some uninterrupted "me time." Or simply let the battery die now and again to remind yourself how to live "unconnected."

- **Zone out.** Download an app and listen to a guided meditation or motivational story. Clearing your mind and focusing on just one thing can feel like a hard reboot for your system.

- **Schedule time to panic.** This was especially helpful for me during COVID-19. Instead of letting the what-ifs keep me up all night, every night, I relegated my "worry time" to fifteen minutes a day. Try using one of your morning walks (or maybe an evening soak in the tub) as a time to ponder the worst-case scenarios, then commit to leaving them behind when time is up.

- **Learn to focus on yourself.** You can't ignore your own needs and spend your entire day caring for the needs of others and expect to be your best self. You will have nothing left and will burn out. Start small to practice making room for you.

Back-to-basics food solutions

Did you know we make more than two hundred decisions a day—just about food? If you're already feeling overwhelmed, it's time to simplify. This book will teach you how to streamline your food choices to focus on ones that will boost your energy, nourish your immune system, and support your mood, focus, and sleep. The meal plans help you establish healthy habits, reignite your flame, and banish burnout.

- **Plan your meals (but leave some wiggle room).** Each chapter includes a meal plan devoted to a specific area of burnout, from focus to sleep, mood to immunity. You can follow these plans to eat better, reduce food waste, and cut down on decision fatigue. If strict plans stress you out, you can work these recipes into your week in your own way, in between Taco Tuesday and Pizza Friday. You can also swap things as you see fit between cooking recipes (when you have the time and interest) and the grab 'n' go or nearly no-cook dinner ideas.

- **Prioritize plants.** This plan is heavy on the plants, from fruits and vegetables to nuts, seeds, pulses, and whole grains. Not only do you get plenty of fiber (provided *only* by plants), but you also get a host of other essential nutrients and phytochemicals. You'll learn all about the benefits of a plant-centric diet—and why it can be so helpful when you're dealing with burnout.

- **And make room for quality protein, too.** You'll notice three exceptions to the "eat plants" part of the plan: eggs, dairy, and seafood. Why? All three are packed with protein and boast specific health benefits. Eggs are an inexpensive, high-quality source of protein, and the yolks provide choline for brain health. Dairy offers calcium, potassium, and vitamin D to boost your mood and support bone health (although fortified dairy alternatives are fine, too!). Seafood packs in protein along with DHA and EPA omega-3 fats for heart and brain health as well as mood regulation.

- **Embrace healthy fats.** Thankfully, we've moved beyond the fat-free craze, when everything from dairy to baked goods was stripped of fats—both the bad ones and the good ones. Fat is an essential macronutrient that plays numerous roles in the body, from insulating cells and producing hormones to helping absorb vitamins A, D, E, and K. You also need to eat sufficient amounts of healthy fats to keep your hair, skin, and nails healthy and supple. The meals in this book focus on "good" fats—mostly unsaturated ones and omega-3s.

- **Focus on whole (or minimally processed) foods.** Many of the (ultra) processed foods sold to us as time savers are really more like high-interest loans. These shortcuts can contribute to our burnout, so replace them with whole foods that help nourish your body instead of depleting it. My meal plans and recipes also include nutrient-dense, minimally processed foods like canned fish, microwavable whole grains, and jarred minced garlic. I know making pasta sauce from scratch and soaking your beans overnight are simply not options when you're frazzled. Many of these foods are also budget-friendly, which reduces stress as well.

- **Find your balance in the kitchen.** We all have different interest levels, skill sets, and availability when it comes to cooking. If baking sourdough bread on the weekend is your way of recharging, that's great. However, if cooking generally adds stress to your life and a midday hike is more your speed, grab a yogurt with granola and hit the trails.

- **Limit added sugar, caffeine, and alcohol.** No food is off-limits, but certain ones can deplete energy and make stress worse when you overdo them. The plans I share will help you cut back on three that can have the most negative impact on your health. Your tolerance for and relationship with this trio can also change throughout life. For example, as you'll learn in chapter 6, caffeine can have a greater impact on your ability to sleep as you age.

  The added sugar in this plan is usually in the form of unrefined options like honey or maple syrup. Naturally sweet fruit is often used as well—think dates, grapes, ripe bananas, and 100 percent pomegranate juice.

More about plants

While the food plan in this book is plant-centric, if you enjoy red meat, chicken, or other animal products, it's fine to include them sometimes. Animal products contain many nutrients that are key to beating burnout, including heme iron, protein, and vitamin B$_{12}$. We don't focus on those in this book because it's probably already easy enough for you to incorporate those foods into your diet.

It's on the plant side of things where most of us fall short. For example, 95 percent of U.S. adults and kids aren't getting enough fiber. And when it comes to getting enough fruits and vegetables, only about one in ten adults hits the mark.

Eating a mostly plant-based diet can offer all sorts of benefits, including.

- Weight loss or maintenance

- Lower risk of heart disease

- Lower risks for certain types of cancer

- Lower rates of cognitive decline

- Lower rates of type 2 diabetes

Whether you're a vegan, a meat lover, or you prefer to mix it up, the recipes in this book will give you more plant-centric options to add to your recipe repertoire, along with the nutrients you need to replenish your body and mind.

In chapter 7 you'll find nourishing and delicious plant-centric recipes, of which more than half are vegan or offer vegan options. And they won't take you loads of time to cook (that would be counterproductive in a book on burnout!). More than half of the recipes take thirty minutes or less, and more than a third take fifteen minutes or less.

Fiber 101

Another advantage of eating (mostly) plants? They're the only source of fiber! According to the U.S. Department of Agriculture, adults in the United States consume only about half of the recommended intake for fiber. Fiber plays an important role in weight management, heart health, blood sugar regulation, and proper digestion.

Fiber cannot be digested or absorbed by the body and comes in two basic forms: soluble and insoluble.

- **Soluble fiber** dissolves in water, forming a gel-like substance that passes through the digestive system. Soluble fiber has been shown to help lower cholesterol levels in the body, which can help reduce the risk of heart disease. You can find soluble fiber in foods such as oats, beans, peas, apples, and citrus fruits.

- **Insoluble fiber** does not dissolve in water and adds bulk to help the movement of material through the digestive system. This can help prevent constipation or struggles with bowel movements. Insoluble fiber can be found in foods like whole grains, nuts, legumes, cauliflower, and potatoes.

By eating a diet that's rich in plants, like the one you'll see throughout this book, you can easily meet your fiber goals.

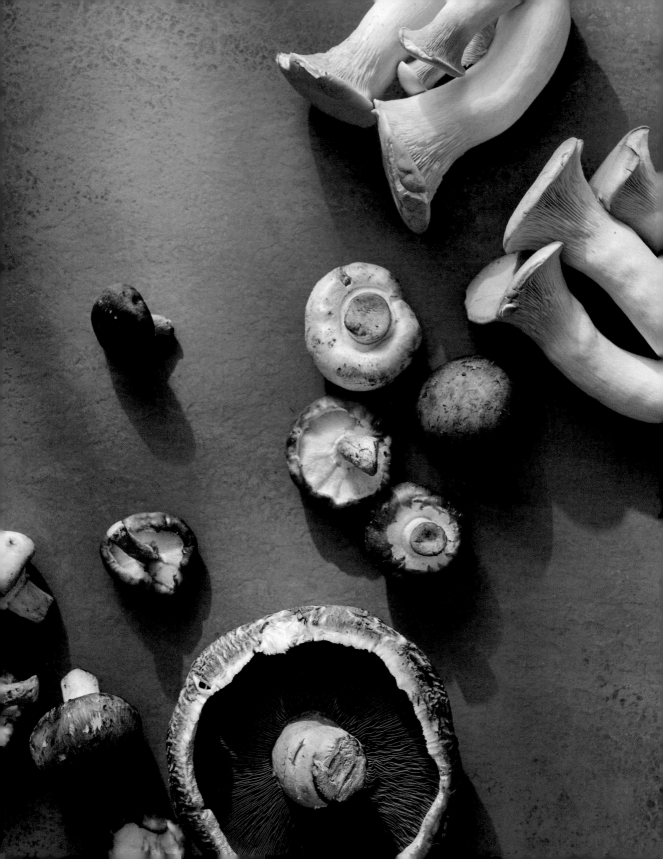

What About Vitamin Supplements?

When it comes to getting the essential nutrients your body needs to stay healthy, food should come first, according to the 2020 Dietary Guidelines for Americans. However, a multivitamin or other supplement can help fill in the gaps.

Depending on their diet and unique needs, some women may benefit from a specific supplement, such as an algae-based omega-3 supplement with EPA/DHA (if you don't eat fatty fish), or perhaps a vitamin D_3, calcium, iron, or vitamin B_{12} supplement.

But before you pop any pill—even a vitamin—you should check with your registered dietitian or other health care provider. You can overdo it on some nutrients, and supplements can also interact with medications.

You need to reach adequate intakes of nutrients to reap the benefits and avoid deficiency symptoms, but more of a nutrient doesn't necessarily mean more of a benefit. Oftentimes too much can have undesirable or even toxic results.

Kitchen-simplification plan

To relieve stress, start by simplifying one of the most anxiety-producing rooms of the house: the kitchen. I know, I know. While I don't want to create more work for you, especially when you're dealing with burnout, I do want to make cooking and preparing food a less stressful, more enjoyable experience.

Take a quick look around your kitchen. Feeling stressed already? Maybe your shelves are stocked with food, but you feel like there's never anything to eat. Your pots and pans are mismatched. Your storage containers never have lids that fit. This makes meal prep, cooking, and cleanup a pain. Streamlining and organizing your kitchen can help. And if you're like me, seeing a project through to the end feels rewarding (even when you really should be doing something else).

Start with just one cupboard or drawer at a time to avoid getting overwhelmed. First get rid of the obvious things that are worn out and broken. Put tools and equipment that work but that you don't use into a box to donate. Keep a list of things that you need to buy or replace. Clean everything, put away what you're keeping, and move to the next cupboard or drawer.

Declutter your pantry, freezer, and fridge, too. Toss out things that are expired and donate unopened products that aren't your favorite (or the best for you).

food staple shopping list

Now that your kitchen is cleaned out and organized, it's time to stock your pantry and freezer with healthy staples to help you quickly pull together nourishing meals.

    With these staples in stock, when you plan for your week, you will only have to replenish fresh ingredients (eggs, dairy or dairy alternatives, produce, and herbs) and ingredients you need to make specific recipes.

Canned & dry goods

- **Cereals and granolas** (high-fiber, low-sugar)
- **Diced or whole peeled tomatoes** (no salt added)
- **Dried and canned beans and lentils** (no salt added)
- **Dried fruit** (no sugar added)
- **Fermented foods** (kimchi, pickles, sauerkraut, etc.)
- **Fish packed in water or olive oil** (tuna, salmon, sardines, etc.)
- **Flours** (all-purpose, almond, whole-wheat, etc.)
- **Low-sodium soups and broths**
- **Nutritional yeast**
- **Nuts and seeds** (store in the refrigerator or freezer for a longer shelf life)
- **Nut and seed butters** (without added sugar)
- **Whole grains** (oats, quinoa, whole-grain pasta, etc.)

Condiments, oils & vinegars

- **Classic condiments** (ketchup, mustard, mayonnaise, etc.)
- **Healthy oils** (avocado oil, extra-virgin olive oil, sunflower oil, etc.)
- **Hot sauces**
- **Honey**
- **Jam or preserves** (100% fruit-sweetened and no-sugar-added)
- **Olives**
- **Pure maple syrup**
- **Salsas** (fruit salsa, salsa verde, tomato-based salsa, etc.)
- **Sauces** (tomato sauce, curry sauce, pesto, etc.)
- **Soy sauce or tamari** (reduced-sodium)
- **Vinegars** (red wine, balsamic, apple cider, etc.)

Frozen foods

- **Beans and peas** (edamame, green peas, lima beans, etc.)
- **Burger patties and meatballs** (plant-based or turkey)
- **Fish fillets and shrimp** (without breading or seasoning)
- **Frozen fruit** (without added sugar)
- **Frozen vegetables** (without sauce)
- **Pizzas** (whole-grain or cauliflower crust)
- **Tortillas** (corn or wheat)
- **Whole grains** (microwavable brown rice, whole-grain waffles, etc.)

Spices & seasonings

- **Cocoa powder** (unsweetened)
- **Dark chocolate** (at least 70% cocoa)
- **Dried herbs** (basil, dill, rosemary, etc.)
- **Extracts** (pure vanilla extract, almond extract, etc.)
- **Spices** (cayenne pepper, ground cinnamon, turmeric, etc.)

Teas

- **Herbal teas** (chamomile, peppermint, ginger, etc.)
- **Teas** (black, green, oolong, etc.)

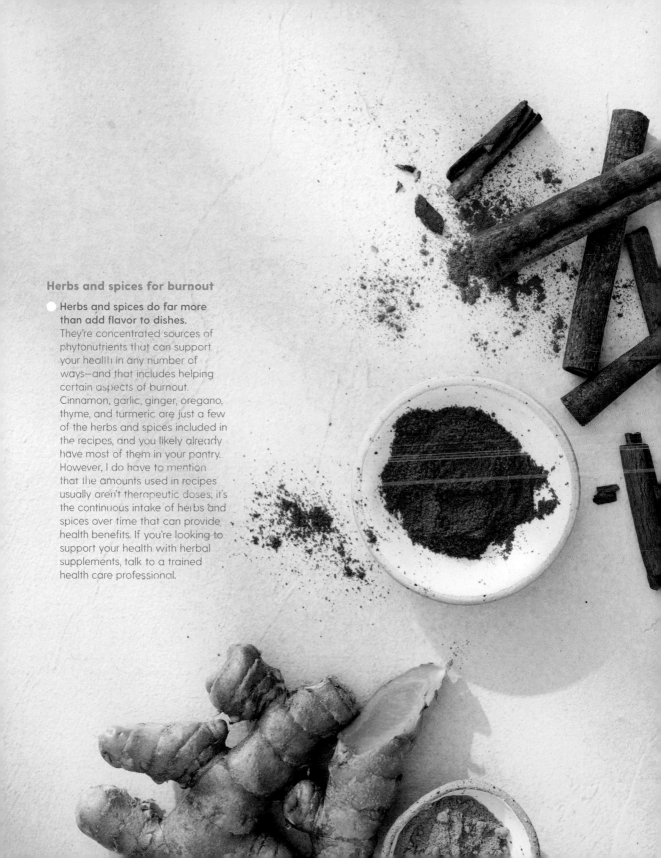

Herbs and spices for burnout

Herbs and spices do far more than add flavor to dishes. They're concentrated sources of phytonutrients that can support your health in any number of ways—and that includes helping certain aspects of burnout. Cinnamon, garlic, ginger, oregano, thyme, and turmeric are just a few of the herbs and spices included in the recipes, and you likely already have most of them in your pantry. However, I do have to mention that the amounts used in recipes usually aren't therapeutic doses; it's the continuous intake of herbs and spices over time that can provide health benefits. If you're looking to support your health with herbal supplements, talk to a trained health care professional.

Budget and Time Savers

Sometimes saving time is of the utmost importance; other times, it's all about that bottom line and pinching pennies. At the grocery store, I work to find a balance, for my budget and my workload in the kitchen. Here are my top picks to save time and money:

- **Avocados:** A must-have to add creaminess and healthy fats, but they can be costly when you don't have a tree in your yard. Buy them when they're on sale. Let ripen, cut in half, peel, wrap tightly, and freeze.

- **Barley:** The "pearled" version cooks up in half the time of other whole grains. Its prebiotic fiber helps keep gut bacteria healthy. It's cheaper than quinoa and has a chewier texture.

- **Canned beans:** Stock up on all kinds and colors for soups, salads, and dips. Beans are tops for the type of fiber that keeps gut-brain communications in harmony.

- **Canned tomatoes:** Diced, pureed, and paste should all have a place in your cupboard for making a quick sauce, pasta topping, or soup. The lycopene that gives tomatoes their red color helps protect against various diseases.

- **Dark leafy greens:** Prewashed salad and cooking greens save time and effort. Just take out of the clamshell or bag and add to your salad, soup, smoothie, or skillet. If you have the time and want to save some money, buy heads of lettuce and bunches of kale, then clean and store them as soon as you get home. (You can even freeze extras to add to smoothies or soups!)

- **Eggs:** These are just about the best-quality protein in the easiest form to use for the least amount of money per gram of protein. Eggs also provide choline for memory and mood support.

- **Fatty fish (canned or frozen):** Fresh fish can be expensive—and might spoil before you can use it. The frozen and canned versions are also packed with mood-boosting omega-3 fatty acids and are easy to use in recipes.

- **Frozen fruit:** Fresh berries aren't always in season and can perish quickly, and tropical fruits are costly when you don't live in the tropics. Thankfully frozen fruit is picked at peak ripeness, then frozen so you can affordably enjoy it year-round.

- **Frozen veggies:** Pick your favorites and stock up. Frozen veggies have come so far, and you can get all your favorites for less. Plus, they're a lifesaver on nights when you can't bear to chop anything!

- **Greek yogurt:** Yogurt (even plant-based versions) is versatile and packed with nutrition. Traditional Greek yogurt has more protein and less sugar than regular yogurt, and the thick consistency makes it a great swap for sour cream.

- **Green herb sauces:** Pick up a container of pesto, chimichurri, or salsa verde to quickly flavor up meals all week. They're packed with nutrient-rich fresh herbs, and you don't have to do the rinsing and chopping. Keep a couple on hand to stir into soup, flavor dips, drizzle on bowls, or turn into tasty salad dressing.

- **Microwavable whole grains:** Perfectly cooked in three minutes or less, microwavable steam-in-the-bag varieties of whole grains in your pantry or freezer make for a high-fiber side dish or veggie bowl base. Options include organic brown rice, quinoa, and flavored bean-and-whole-grain blends.

- **Nut butters:** Good ol' peanut butter is affordable and tasty, but branch out and try others like almond, sunflower seed, and cashew. Beyond fixing PB&Js for the kids, you can use nut butters to make creamy sauces, drizzle them on oatmeal, or eat them off a spoon for a snack. They provide plant-based protein, healthy fats, and fiber to keep gut bacteria happy. Choose natural versions with no added oils or sugars.

- **Oats:** Whether steel cut, old-fashioned rolled, or quick-cooking, oats are packed with nutrients to start your day. They're awesome for overnight oatmeal, cook up pretty quickly for a hot breakfast, and make a delicious and crunchy topping when baked.

- **Ready-cut vegetables:** Yeah, you'll pay a bit more for them, but this is where that time-versus-money decision comes in. The less time you spend peeling butternut squash or zoodling zucchini, the more time you have for you. Look for frozen versions to save money.

- **Refrigerated or frozen minced garlic and ginger:** These flavor boosters retain their nutrition and stay fresh for months. I always have a jar of each on hand for quick meals—and it saves time because I don't have to mince or puree anything. Crushed frozen options are also available.

- **Sparkling water:** The festive fizziness of sparkling water makes you feel good and keeps your body hydrated. Squeeze in some citrus—lemon, lime, or tangerine. Treat yourself to a seltzer in place of a glass of wine or can of soda. Or for those nights when you really want (or need) a glass of wine, make it a wine spritzer with half sparkling water.

20 nearly no-cook dinner ideas

With a fully stocked, organized kitchen, healthy meals truly can come together in minutes. While chapter 7 is packed with nourishing and delicious recipes, there are those nights when cooking is simply not going to happen! Don't force it. You need to lighten your load to focus on wellness, which often means doing less. That's where these nearly no-cook dinner ideas come in. These are quick-assembly dinners that make use of the pantry and freezer staples from your list above. (Be sure to read packaging for specific preparation instructions.)

1. **Salmon Supper**
   Roast or pan-grill a frozen salmon fillet; serve with microwavable brown rice and a mixed green side salad dressed with lemon and olive oil; sprinkle everything with sliced almonds.

2. **Plant-Based Burger & Fries**
   Prepare a fresh or frozen plant-based burger; serve on a whole-grain bun with lettuce, tomato, and your favorite condiments; serve with oven-baked frozen sweet potato fries or a microwave-baked sweet potato.

3. **Grilled Cheese & Tomato Soup**
   Lightly sprinkle thin-sliced whole-grain bread with part-skim mozzarella, form a sandwich, brush with olive oil, and toast in a skillet; simmer store-bought organic tomato soup to serve alongside.

4. **Mexican Salad Bowl**
   On mixed salad greens, arrange drained canned black beans, thawed frozen corn, sliced avocado, sliced grape tomatoes, shredded Monterey jack cheese, and a few tortilla chips; dress with salsa verde.

5. **Peanut Noodles with Edamame**
   Toss cooked linguine with cooked shelled edamame, sliced red bell pepper, and bottled Asian peanut sauce; top with fresh cilantro or scallions, crushed red pepper flakes, and lime wedges.

6. **Savory Oatmeal**
   Prepare oatmeal with vegetable broth; stir in fresh baby spinach and sliced sun-dried tomatoes; sprinkle with goat cheese or top with a fried egg; serve with lemon wedges.

7. **Lentil Soup & Crusty Bread**
   Simmer store-bought organic carrot-lentil soup or other vegetarian lentil soup; top with a dollop of prepared pesto; serve with a piece of crusty whole-grain baguette and a small bunch of grapes.

8. **Pizza Night**
   Bake frozen vegetarian cauliflower-crust pizza; serve with sautéed fresh zucchini coins; enjoy with fresh watermelon or other melon.

9. **Quick Bean & Cheese Quesadilla**
   Top whole wheat tortillas with shredded Monterey jack cheese and drained canned black beans; fold in half; toast in a hot skillet; top with prepared guacamole.

10. **Easy Tuna Soft Tacos**
Fill warm corn or wheat tortillas with drained canned flaked tuna; top with slaw mix (or shredded cabbage), prepared guacamole, store-bought pico de gallo or salsa, and fresh cilantro.

11. **Pesto Pasta Salad**
Cook farfalle or rotini pasta, rinse with cold water or toss with ice, then drain; toss cooled pasta with prepared pesto, fresh baby spinach, chopped walnuts, and a squirt of lemon; serve with a boiled or deviled egg.

12. **Mediterranean Snack Board with Veggies**
On a wooden cutting board or a platter, arrange raw carrots, cherry tomatoes, sliced cucumber, hummus, olives, figs, feta cheese, and fresh whole-grain pita wedges.

13. **Shrimp Stir-Fry**
Stir-fry peeled deveined shrimp, fresh pre-sliced mushrooms, and frozen veggies (carrots, broccoli, cauliflower, etc.) in sunflower oil in a wok or large sauté pan; toss with bottled natural stir-fry sauce to heat; serve over microwavable ancient grains.

14. **Spaghetti & "Meatballs" & More**
Prepare fresh or frozen plant-based meatballs and cook spaghetti; toss meatballs and spaghetti with store-bought marinara sauce and fresh baby kale or spinach until greens are wilted; sprinkle with nutritional yeast flakes.

15. **Lentil Salad Bowl**
Toss drained canned lentils with chopped fresh flat-leaf parsley and mint, quartered grape tomatoes, and thinly sliced scallions; season with sea salt and garlic powder; dress with lemon juice and olive oil; sprinkle with optional feta cheese.

16. **Soup & Sides**
Simmer store-bought organic sweet potato soup; serve with sides of microwavable brown rice and steamed frozen broccoli with tamari or soy sauce to taste; pair with pistachios or peanuts.

17. **Savory Greek Yogurt Bowl**
Serve plain Greek yogurt in a bowl topped with diced English cucumber and olive oil, sprinkle with sea salt, pomegranate arils, and fresh mint leaves; serve with multigrain pita chips and a lemon wedge.

18. **"Chicken & Waffles"**
Prepare plant-based breaded "chicken" strips for nuggets; prepare frozen wholegrain waffles; serve "chicken" on waffles and drizzle lightly with maple syrup; pair with peaches or berries.

19. **Mediterranean Snack Board with Fruit**
On a wooden cutting board or a platter, arrange grapes, orange wedges, dates, goat cheese, pistachios, radishes, canned sardines in olive oil, and flatbreads or crusty whole-grain baguette slices.

20. **Curry Tuna Salad Wrap**
Stir drained canned tuna with mayonnaise, curry powder, diced red onion, raisins, and fresh cilantro; wrap in a whole-grain tortilla with mixed baby greens and a squirt of lime juice.

About the recipes in this book

The satisfying, nutrient-packed recipes in chapter 7 are designed so you can easily choose what works best for you. Recipes are marked:

Vegan	No Added Sugar
Vegetarian	Kid-Friendly
One-Dish Meal	Great for Leftovers
Gluten-Free	Smart Freezer Meal
Nut-Free	15 Minutes or Less
Dairy-Free	30 Minutes or Less

More than half of the recipes in this book are ready in thirty minutes or less, and many are ready in fifteen minutes or less. There are also some recipes that are a bit more complex for those who love to cook and want a recipe beyond overnight oats; these meals are also great for the beginner who wants a special-occasion recipe. For example, the Shaved Asparagus and Potato Frittata on page 108 is perfect if you're a newbie chef and want something special to cook for a family brunch that is both healthy and sure to please a crowd.

For additional ease, freezer meals are recipes that you can batch cook and then freeze in individual portions to help your future self have a healthy meal ready in minutes.

Each recipe has an optional "supercharger" ingredient (like chia seeds, coconut flakes, or fresh basil). This is an ingredient that you can add to elevate the nutrient profile and taste, but one you can omit if you don't want to make a special trip to the store or simply don't like it. While the superchargers do offer additional nutrients, I don't want to pretend that the portions are large enough for you to garner health benefits from using them in just one recipe. The idea is rather that you may discover you like a wider variety of nutrient-dense foods or learn new ways of incorporating them into your diet. Then, over time, as you start to consume your preferred superchargers on a regular basis, you will reap the health benefits.

The recipes include basic nutrition information and indicate whether each recipe is an "excellent" or "good" source of different nutrients. Excellent sources provide at least 20 percent of the daily value of a particular vitamin or nutrient per serving, while good sources provide 10 to 19 percent of the daily value.

If an ingredient is noted as optional, such as a supercharger, it is not included in the nutrition information; however, I do tell you what additional nutrients the supercharger would provide.

About the meal plans in this book

These meal plans are not meant to be followed exactly as written; however, you are certainly welcome to do that if it cuts down on decision fatigue! (Yes, that's a real thing; you'll learn all about it in chapter 5). Rather, the meal plan is meant to serve as inspiration. It's intended to help you see at a glance how your meals might look throughout the week. Then you can pick and choose according to your time and preferences.

The snacks are a good example of this. While I suggest three specific snacks each day, you can swap out the snacks. In fact, to make it easier, refer to the list of suggested snacks (both recipes and grab 'n' go) at the end of each meal plan.

The meal plans are designed for you to help your future self: dinner recipes are usually repurposed as tasty leftovers for lunch the following day.

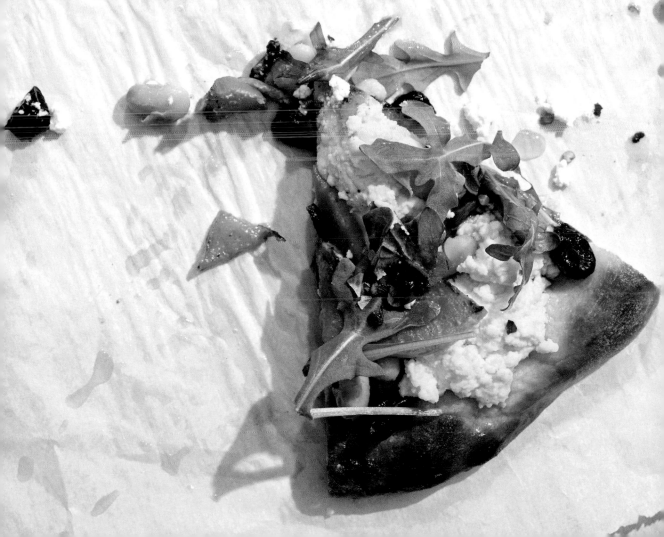

1-week burnout-busting meal plan

Your meal plan for this week will ease you into a new style of eating, so it's a little different from the others, which are focused on a single aspect of burnout or an ailment. This week's meal plan instead centers around the idea of embracing a core group of nourishing foods that take as little time and energy as possible to prepare. You'll encounter one-dish dinners, freezer meals, tasty leftovers, and healthy store-bought foods to help you get the nutrition you and your family need—for a lot less effort!

And for those nights when you "can't even" deal with making dinner, simply swap the suggested recipe for one of the twenty nearly no-cook dinner ideas on pages 38–39.

Monday

Breakfast
Yogurt with strawberries and cinnamon

Snack
Banana with peanut butter

Lunch
Store-bought minestrone soup, whole-grain crackers, and an orange

Snack
Store-bought sea-salt-and-olive-oil popcorn

Dinner
Mediterranean Eggplant Hummus Bowl (page 130) with Fresh Herb Hummus (page 131) and whole wheat pita (Tip: Make extra hummus to enjoy throughout the week)

Snack
Five-Ingredient Chocolate Chip Banana Oat Bites (page 207) (Tip: Make extra to enjoy throughout the week)

Note
Freeze bananas for soft serve tomorrow

Tuesday

Breakfast
Five-Ingredient Chocolate Chip Banana Oat Bites (leftover)

Snack
Apple and cheese

Lunch
Fresh Herb Hummus (leftover) in a veggie wrap

Snack
Green Tea Soft Serve (page 216) (Tip: Make extra to enjoy throughout the week)

Dinner
Raw Asparagus and Edamame Salad with Sesame-Lime Dressing (page 195) with wild rice

Snack
Dark chocolate and walnuts

Wednesday

Breakfast
Sprouted whole-grain avocado toast

Snack
Fresh Herb Hummus (leftover) and bell pepper strips

Lunch
Raw Asparagus and Edamame Salad with Sesame-Lime Dressing (leftover) (Tip: Supercharge it with a hard-boiled egg)

Snack
Five-Ingredient Chocolate Chip Oat Bites (leftover)

Dinner
Simple Salmon Burgers with Grape Salsa (page 144)

Snack
Peanut Butter Stuffed Dates (page 211)

Thursday

- **Breakfast**
  Blueberry Cacao Smoothie
  (page 159)
- **Snack**
  Whole-food snack bar
- **Lunch**
  Simple Salmon Burger patty
  (leftover) over a green salad
- **Snack**
  Green Tea Soft Serve (leftover)
- **Dinner**
  Kimchi, Corn, and Scallion Fried
  Rice (page 136)
- **Snack**
  Store-bought sea-salt-and-
  olive-oil popcorn

Friday

- **Breakfast**
  High-fiber cereal with milk and
  peaches
- **Snack**
  Store-bought roasted chickpea
  snack
- **Lunch**
  Kimchi, Corn, and Scallion Fried
  Rice (leftover)
- **Snack**
  Yogurt with berries
- **Dinner**
  Ultimate Caprese Salad
  Flatbread (page 123)
- **Snack**
  Pumpkin Spice Almond Butter
  Balls (page 212)

Saturday

- **Breakfast**
  Smashed Chickpea Artichoke
  Scramble with Sun-Dried
  Tomatoes (page 114)
- **Snack**
  Pumpkin Spice Almond Butter
  Balls (leftover)
- **Lunch**
  Ultimate Caprese Salad
  Flatbread (leftover)
- **Snack**
  Green Tea Soft Serve (leftover)
- **Dinner**
  Zucchini and Black Bean
  Chilaquiles Skillet (page 143)
- **Snack**
  Grapes and cheese

Sunday

- **Breakfast**
  Fluffy Oat Pancakes with Pears
  (page 105)
- **Snack**
  Dates and peanuts
- **Lunch**
  Plant-based burger with a
  green salad
- **Snack**
  Pumpkin Spice Almond Butter
  Balls (leftover)
- **Dinner**
  One-Pot Thai Red Curry
  (page 171) (Tip: Make extra to
  enjoy throughout the week)
- **Snack**
  100% frozen fruit bar

SUGGESTED SNACKS + SWEETS

Let's Get Cookin'	Grab 'n' Go
Green Tea Soft Serve (page 216)	Green tea and pistachios
Fresh Herb Hummus (page 131) with veggies	Store-bought hummus with veggies
Five-Ingredient Chocolate Chip–Banana Oat Bites (page 207)	Banana with peanut butter
"Cheesy" Lemon Pepper Popcorn (page 203)	Store-bought sea-salt-and-olive-oil popcorn
Peanut Butter Stuffed Dates (page 211)	Dates and peanuts
Pumpkin Spice Almond Butter Balls (page 212)	Whole-food snack bar
Fudgy Avocado Walnut Brownies (page 217)	Dark chocolate and walnuts
Calming Vanilla Lavender Latte (page 160)	Herbal tea and yogurt with berries
Blueberry Cacao Smoothie (page 159)	Dark chocolate and blueberries
Mango Beet Ice Pops (page 215)	100% frozen fruit bar

chapter 3

improve mood

because
fake smiles
don't feel good

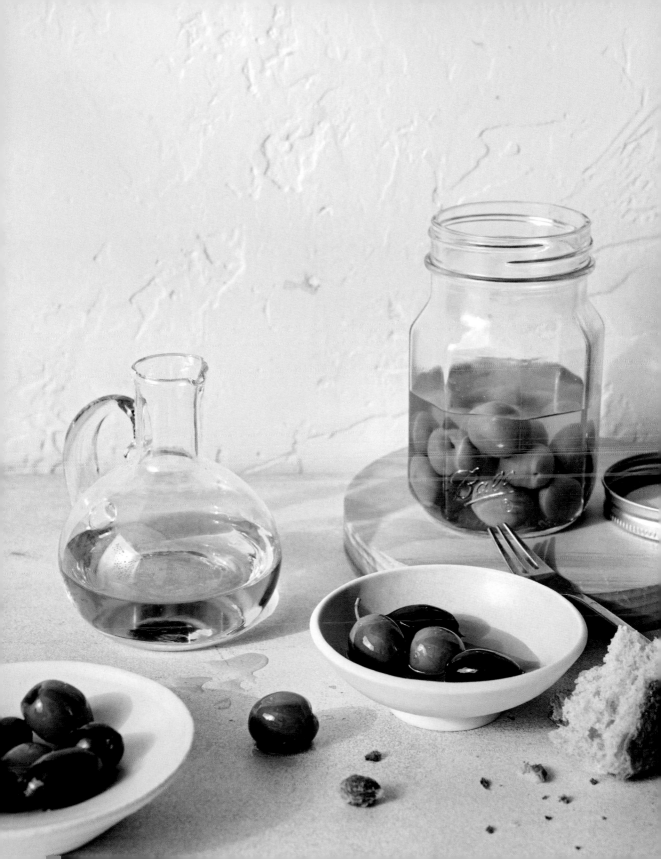

Me: What could possibly go wrong?
Anxiety: I made a list!

—Anonymous

Does it feel like everyone you know is dealing with something big emotionally, yourself included? Does it feel harder than usual to maintain a positive attitude? Are you ready to yell, scream, or snap at the next person who asks you for something? Are you feeling "done"?

You are not alone. And you're not imagining this.

Burnout, anxiety, and depression

Burnout doesn't exist in a vacuum. So that means we're not only exhausted—we're also anxious. Or we're depressed. Research has found a "significant" association between burnout and both anxiety and depression. (As if we didn't have enough to worry about!) There is but one bright light: burnout usually teams up with anxiety *or* depression, but not both at the same time.

Anxiety is your body's way of protecting you during difficult and stressful situations. In small doses, it does what it's supposed to: it keeps you safe. But when you are constantly under stress and your body doesn't get a chance to reset itself from fight-or-flight mode back into rest-and-digest mode, then you end up with anxiety, which has a lot in common with burnout.

Anxiety and burnout are a classic "chicken or egg" situation. Researchers aren't sure whether being prone to anxiety also makes you prone to burning out, or whether burning out makes you anxious, but the exact relationship isn't so important. If you're feeling these feelings, know that there's hope—and you're not imagining any of it.

How hormones affect our mood

How many times have you expressed a feeling, only to be met with: "You're so hormonal"?

Yep. You are. We all are. When you're burned out, your hormones are not in balance and are often trying desperately to find equilibrium. Of course you might feel like your fuse is short or you're about to cry at any moment.

You've already read how stress and burnout impact your cortisol and adrenaline levels. But there are so many other ways that your hormones can impact your mood. Our female hormones may even be the reason why we experience mood disorders disproportionately compared to males after puberty.

PMS

Premenstrual syndrome (PMS) isn't an insult to be lobbed at a woman who's emotional. It's a real, sometimes life-altering group of symptoms that affects 90 percent of women in the week or two before they start their periods. It's most likely to impact women who are in their thirties but can happen at any age.

Beyond the bloating, breast tenderness, headaches, and cravings, PMS can cause moodiness. And if you already have burnout, depression, or anxiety, PMS may make those conditions worse.

Your cycle

As you may know, our two main reproductive hormones are estrogen and progesterone. Each has specific roles and naturally fluctuates throughout the menstrual cycle (and life cycle). Here's a quick refresher on what happens hormonally during your cycle:

Day 1: Your period starts. Estrogen is low, which can cause depression or irritability.

Days 2–4: Your period continues, and you might keep feeling crummy.

Days 5–8: Estrogen rises, which boosts feel-good endorphins. You start to feel like yourself again, with more energy and less anxiety.

Day 14: Estrogen levels peak with ovulation. You might feel like your best—sexiest, funniest, and smartest—self around this time.

Days 15–23: Progesterone starts to rise.

Days 24–28: Both progesterone and estrogen drop, which can cause mood changes. This is the time when PMS happens.

Menopause

During menopause, as your body slows and eventually ceases your menstrual cycle, your levels of progesterone and estrogen can be all over the place. No wonder so many women feel like menopause is an emotional roller coaster.

From night sweats and anxiety to fatigue and changes in libido and bone density, menopause and the years leading up to it (called perimenopause) can be a time of emotional turmoil. Researchers working on the ten-year Study of Women's Health Across the Nation found that women were at a greater risk for depressive symptoms (and depression) during and mostly after this transitional period—and they found four other long-term studies with similar results.

This depression wasn't situational, meaning a depression that happens as a result of a stressful life event. It was related to a chemical or hormonal shift in the brain. And women who were younger and had a negative view of aging and menopause were more likely to report feeling depressed.

Pregnancy and postpartum depression

Your hormones also change drastically throughout pregnancy and into the "fourth trimester." Beyond the sleep deprivation and being tethered to your beautiful and perfect (but oh-so-demanding) new baby, your body is also adjusting to not growing another life. You're bound to experience ups and downs.

Postpartum depression is far more common than we once thought, affecting one in nine new moms. It's important that we talk about this condition out in the open, without shame. We have enough to worry about when it comes to parenting! Within one day of giving birth, your estrogen and progesterone go from their highest peak to their pre-pregnancy levels. That's a huge change basically overnight. It's like a turbo version of the change that happens during your menstrual cycle!

And when you couple all those natural changes with sleep deprivation, often too-short parental leaves, and all the other work you have to do, it's no wonder that mothering can lead to mood changes and burnout!

After her second daughter was born, Kimball felt pressure to be the primary provider in every way—to her children, her staff, her spouse, and her community. Her need to be in charge morphed into a compulsion. "Everything had to be perfect," she says. "My first daughter was a toddler then and ate the cleanest, healthiest everything. The house had to be freakishly clean and tidy. Meanwhile, my newborn wasn't sleeping more than an hour at a time." That's when her burnout was at its worst.

How Five Minutes in Nature Can Boost Your Mood

A study published by the *Journal of Positive Psychology* recently showed that a microdose of Mother Earth—just *five* minutes, to be specific—is all you need to feel, and be, happier and healthier. Here's how the study worked: Two groups of university students were assigned to either five minutes or fifteen minutes of sedentary nature contact (during which they simply sat outside). The study showed that after only *five minutes*, participants in the first group reported improved hedonic (pleasant or pleasurable) and self-transcendent emotions. (Self-transcendence is simply the realization that you are one small part of the greater whole.)

Research into the relationship between time outside and improved health and wellness shows that natural environments promote psychological, emotional, and attentional restoration. Exposure to the great outdoors has been associated with reduced recovery times following surgery, improved health outcomes for a variety of conditions (including cancer and cardiovascular disease), and reduced symptoms of attention-deficit/hyperactivity disorder in children. So next time you're frazzled, fried, or simply feeling on the edge, a simple trot around the block may be all you need.

The brain-gut connection

How many times have you said "I have a gut feeling about this" to describe something you can't explain but fully believe? What was once merely a figure of speech is now proven by science: you can trust your gut to tell you when something is up. Ignore that message, and it'll just keep getting louder and louder and louder.

Maybe you've been going through a hard time—a separation, a monster of a boss, or caring for aging parents. You think you're handling it all, but your digestive system is out of whack. You're snacking too much. You don't have an appetite anymore. Your stomach hurts all the time, for no apparent reason. You've changed your diet. You've ruled out digestive ailments. You've done those awful, restrictive elimination diets. (Been there, tried that. Didn't work.) And yet you still feel off.

These "gut feelings" are examples of how your brain and your gut are directly connected. When you ignore the messages your brain tries to send you, it doesn't give up. It simply goes through another path: the gut-brain axis.

Your gut brain

Each one of us has between 200 and 600 million neurons lining our digestive tract. Your "gut brain"—or enteric nervous system—is directly connected to your actual brain, along with the rest of your central nervous system. Your gut and brain are linked up physically, through all those neurons as well as the vagus nerve.

The primary mediator of your parasympathetic nervous system (that is, your rest-and-digest system), the vagus nerve is in charge of getting you to a state of relaxation—and keeping you there. You can think of it as your air-traffic controller, helping to regulate all your major bodily functions. Breathing, heart rate, digestion, and even how you take in, process, and make meaning of your experiences are all directly related to the vagus nerve.

When we're stressed, burned out, or reeling from an emotional crisis, our vagus nerve can't send or receive signals as well, which can also impact our gut health. Research connects reduced "vagal tone" (or lowered function) to conditions like Crohn's disease and irritable bowel syndrome.

Vagal Breathing Technique

Imagine yourself filling up the lower part of your lungs, just above your belly button, like a balloon and then exhaling slowly. (It can help to put a hand on your belly to feel your breath and get the hang of this different movement.) This diaphragmatic breathing, a proven way to stimulate the vagus nerve, may help to explain why yoga or meditation can leave you feeling brand new.

One of the easiest ways to practice vagal breathing is with a 4:8 ratio—four seconds of inhalation followed by an eight-second exhalation. Be sure to inhale through your nose for fuller, deeper breaths that stimulate the lower lungs and distribute more oxygen to the body. (Mouth and chest breathing actually stimulate the upper lungs, which triggers the sympathetic nerve receptors and cause us to hyperventilate.) Exhale through pursed lips as you count to eight, which increases resistance in your airways and helps them to stay open during exhalation. Breathe, release, and repeat any time you're in need of an intentional mental recess.

Aromatherapy: Boost Your Mood with Happy Scents

Aromatherapy uses essential oils from plants as a way to improve physical, mental, and spiritual well-being. Each plant's essential oil has a different makeup, which means each plant affects the body differently. Think lavender for sleep, rosemary for focus, and peppermint for energy during exercise. Or grab a bottle of lemon, wild orange, or thyme essential oils, which have been shown to support a positive mood, including in individuals who suffer from depression.

Wild orange is known to boost spirits and has even been shown to reduce anxiety in women during labor, while other citrus blends (featuring combinations of orange, lemon, lime, grapefruit, and bergamot essential oils) have been shown to restore the immune system after it has been suppressed during stressful times. While they can be inhaled directly or applied to the skin with the help of a carrier oil, essential oils are most often inhaled indirectly through diffusion. (Plus, the sound of a diffuser is totally relaxing.)

A healthy mood starts in the kitchen

A healthy gut—and a healthy mood—starts in the kitchen. What you eat can make you feel good—and no, we're not talking about comfort foods. We're talking about good-mood foods. The kind of food that makes you feel happy, less stressed, calmer, or just all-around better after you eat. The same can't be said for a pan of brownies or bag of tortilla chips.

Certain nutrients and certain foods can help you maintain (or create) a healthy gut-brain axis. (You'll get a full list of foods to fight burnout and boost mood later in this chapter.) These feel-good foods can do all sorts of things:

- Counteract the negative effects of stress hormones

- Keep your blood sugar levels more stable (so being "hungry" can't sabotage your day)

- Help your brain make "happy" hormones like serotonin and dopamine

- Feed your microbiome

Your microbiome

The microbiome is the unsung heroine of your gastrointestinal system. Made up of literally trillions of microbes, it is the community of good bacteria that live in your gut—and impact not only how your digestive system functions but how you feel as well.

Your microbiome is like the bouncer of your gut. When the lining of your digestive tract is healthy, and your microbiome is strong and healthy, the good bacteria can control what gets in and out of your gastrointestinal tract. But when you have problems with your gut (or your mood), it's like a venue that's understaffed or over capacity. Those "bouncers" can't keep up. There's hope, though: you can change your bacteria and, in turn, your mood. That's where probiotics and prebiotics come in.

- **Probiotics** are the good bacteria found in certain foods, like yogurt, kefir, fermented vegetables, miso paste, and tempeh, that help keep the healthy bacteria levels in your gut strong. You want more of the good bugs to crowd out the "bad" ones. Good levels of probiotics keep the link between the brain and belly wide open. They may also provide beneficial mood-boosting neurotransmitters like GABA.

- **Prebiotics** feed those good bacteria in your belly. They help your body cope with stress-related shifts in your microbiome and make sure that the healthy bacteria have the fuel they need to keep you healthy. They're found in whole grains, nuts, seeds, fruits, and vegetables.

The food and mood connection

Food and mood are so intricately connected that they've inspired a new area of psychiatry. Nutritional psychiatry examines how what we eat impacts how we feel. As a dietitian who has experienced this connection firsthand, I find it infinitely fascinating that we can empower ourselves to feel better partly (or sometimes entirely) based on what we choose to put on our plate—or leave off! Food can make or break everything from your productivity at work and your mood on any given day to how much energy you have.

This scientific breakthrough, that we finally have proof that food and mood go hand in hand, is huge—but is it really a breakthrough? We've long known that food can influence immunity, risk for certain diseases, and weight. Why is it groundbreaking that it affects feelings?

Australian researchers are looking into how certain diets can be used alongside psychiatric treatments. They did a small but mighty study that was published in the journal *BMC Medicine* in 2017, appropriately called "SMILES." (It stands for Supporting the Modification of lifestyle In Lowered Emotional States.)

All the researchers did was change the diets of sixty-seven people living with depression. Those who ate a more or less Mediterranean diet were 400 percent more likely to say they were in a good mood than those who were in the control group. Both sets of people were able to use medications or therapy as necessary, but the Mediterranean group significantly reduced three of the biggest bad-mood food groups:

refined sugars, refined grains, and processed vegetable oils. The Mediterranean diet consistently comes out on top when it comes to weight loss, heart health, inflammation, and longevity. Now we can add mood and brain health to that list.

Those cultures that live around the Mediterranean Sea eat mostly whole foods. They eat healthy fats, more vegetables than the average American, whole grains in place of processed ones, some fish and seafood, moderate amounts of dairy and red meats, and even some wine and dark chocolate. Two regions in the Mediterranean—Sardinia in Italy and Ikaria in Greece—are even classified as Blue Zones, places where people not only live longer but are also happier and healthier along the way. That diet is similar to what you'll find in this book, though I don't use the same labels. Foods that reignite your passion for living (good mood foods) and the Mediterranean diet overlap, as you'll see.

Want more proof? According to the American Gut Project, the world's largest crowdsourced, citizen science microbiome research project, eating thirty different plants a week can make for a healthier microbiome (and a healthier mood) than eating ten plants or less. There's also evidence that the amount of fruits and vegetables you eat is related to your risk of depression. Basically, eating more of them can improve your mood and mental health. And these plant-based foods also improve life expectancy and quality.

But that doesn't mean you can only eat salads. Fruits and vegetables count, of course, but so do legumes, nuts, seeds, whole grains, and even mushrooms (technically fungi). And as you'll learn in the next sections, plenty of other foods can influence your mood.

Mood-boosting nutrients and foods

When it comes to food, I keep this mantra in mind: *Whole foods make a whole person.* Tempting as it might be to fill the hole that burnout leaves with comforting sugary or salty snacks, those won't help bring you back. The most profound changes happen when we stick with the basics. Eating a variety of foods that are as unprocessed as possible— while still keeping mealtime simple for your sake—is the basis of the plan in this book

Oftentimes, when we talk about nutrition, we associate a single food with a single benefit or nutrient. But that's not how nutrition works—or how your body works. Whole foods, from a fillet of sockeye salmon to a cup of strawberries, contain a host of nutrients, each with its own unique benefits, and they work synergistically within your body. So while I highlight certain foods both in this chapter and throughout the book, they are far from the *only* ones that will benefit your body, your mind—or even your mood. And that's why you don't need to memorize daily values and milligram amounts for each nutrient (trying to do that would burn *anyone* out!).

Instead, you'll learn how certain nutrients— and the categories of foods that contain them—impact your emotional health. This will start to show you how simple nutrition can be, and how choosing whole, unprocessed foods can begin to help you dig your way out of burnout, one meal at a time.

And if you don't have the energy to digest all the nutrient information and food lists just yet, no need to fret. In addition to my more thorough explanations, here is your stress-free, at-a-glance cheat sheet of twenty-five top mood-boosting foods and why they help:

25 mood-boosting foods to include on your grocery list

Apples
antioxidant quercetin for neurotransmitters, vitamin C to help stabilize mood, prebiotic fiber for gut health

Asparagus
vitamin C to help stabilize mood, folate for neurotransmitters, prebiotic fiber for gut health

Avocados
folate for neurotransmitters, magnesium to reduce anxiety, healthy fats for hormones and brain health

Bananas
vitamin B_6 to make serotonin, prebiotic fiber for gut health, vitamin C to help stabilize mood

Bell peppers
vitamin C to help stabilize mood, vitamin B_6 for neurotransmitters

Carrots
vitamin A for mood support, prebiotic fiber for gut health, folate for neurotransmitters

Chia seeds
protein and fiber to stabilize blood sugar levels, calcium to ease PMS and support a healthy mood, iron for energy

Chickpeas
protein and fiber to stabilize blood sugar levels, folate for neurotransmitters, iron for energy, magnesium to reduce anxiety

Dark chocolate
polyphenols and flavonoids to reduce the stress hormone cortisol, magnesium to reduce anxiety

Eggs
choline for energy and a steady mood, B vitamins for managing stress and energy, antioxidant selenium to support a healthy mood

Garlic
prebiotic fiber for gut health, antioxidants for mood support

Green tea
L-theanine for calm, caffeine for energy and mental clarity, antioxidants for mood support

Kimchi
active cultures for a healthy microbiome

Lemons and limes
vitamin C to help stabilize mood, citrus aromas may boost mood

 Lentils
complex carbs for brain food, antioxidant selenium to support a healthy mood, B vitamins for managing stress and energy, iron for energy

 Oats and oatmeal
complex carbs for brain food, magnesium to reduce anxiety, B vitamins for managing stress and energy, prebiotics for gut health

 Olives and olive oil
healthy fats for hormones and brain health

 Oysters
iron for energy, zinc for a healthy mood

 Pistachios
protein and fiber to stabilize blood sugar levels, healthy fats for hormones and brain health, vitamin B_6 to make neurotransmitters

 Pumpkin seeds
healthy fats for hormones and brain health, magnesium to reduce anxiety, zinc for a healthy mood, prebiotics for gut health

 Salmon
protein for a stable mood, omega-3 fats for brain health and mood, vitamins D and B_{12} to support serotonin levels

 Spinach
magnesium to reduce anxiety, folate for neurotransmitters, vitamin C to help stabilize mood

 Strawberries
vitamin C to help stabilize mood, prebiotic fiber for gut health, flavonoids to help regulate mood

 Yogurt
active cultures for a healthy microbiome, calcium to ease PMS and support a healthy mood

 Zucchini
vitamin C to help stabilize mood, magnesium to reduce anxiety, folate for neurotransmitters

While this cheat sheet can help you quickly choose foods to support your mood, see pages 223–31 for a more comprehensive list to help guide your mood-boosting food choices.

1-week mood-boosting meal plan

Above all, this is a book written with real life in mind. I get it: you don't always have the time (or the energy or interest) to cook dinner from scratch. Neither do I. Sometimes I order takeout, use a meal-delivery service, or take shortcuts with prepared ingredients from the supermarket.

Your mood-boosting meal plan offers options for whatever you feel like doing today: Choose from simple, healthy recipe ideas when you feel like cooking. Or pick one of the store-bought shortcuts when you're lacking time or energy.

No matter which path you choose, this meal plan is designed to help out your future self. For example, each dinner recipe in the meal plan is set up to work as a leftover for the following day's lunch. And for those nights when you're not in the mood to cook dinner, no problem! Swap a dinner recipe for one of the twenty nearly no-cook dinner ideas on pages 38–39. It will put a smile on your face in no time!

Monday

Breakfast
Oatmeal with banana and cinnamon

Snack
Green tea and pistachios

Lunch
Whole-grain sourdough toast with sliced avocado, tomato, and feta

Snack
Store-bought sea-salt-and-olive-oil popcorn

Dinner
Cauliflower and Black Bean Chili (page 174)

Snack
Better-Than-Ever Banana Bread (page 209)

Note
Freeze bananas for smoothie tomorrow morning

Tuesday

Breakfast
Pomegranate, Mandarin, and Ginger Smoothie (page 157)

Snack
Store-bought hummus with veggies

Lunch
Cauliflower and Black Bean Chili (leftover)

Snack
Better-Than-Ever Banana Bread (leftover)

Dinner
Poblano and Portobello Tacos (page 125)

Snack
Dates and peanuts

Wednesday

Breakfast
Yogurt with kiwi and almonds

Snack
Better-Than-Ever Banana Bread (leftover)

Lunch
Poblano and Portobello Taco filling (leftover) over a green salad

Snack
Hard-boiled egg and bell pepper strips

Dinner
Sheet-Pan Salmon, Fingerling Potatoes, and Asparagus with Citrus Miso Sauce (page 119)

Snack
Golden Carrot Spice Muffins (page 116)

Thursday

- **Breakfast**
  Golden Carrot Spice Muffin
  (leftover)

- **Snack**
  Hummus Deviled Eggs
  (page 206)

- **Lunch**
  Sheet-Pan Salmon, Fingerling
  Potatoes, and Asparagus with
  Citrus Miso Sauce (leftover)
  made into a Nicoise salad with
  leafy greens, hard-boiled egg,
  and tomatoes

- **Snack**
  Whole-food snack bar

- **Dinner**
  Kimchi, Corn, and Scallion
  Fried Rice (page 136)

- **Snack**
  Dark chocolate and walnuts

Friday

- **Breakfast**
  High-fiber cereal with
  banana and milk

- **Snack**
  Mandarin and pumpkin
  seeds

- **Lunch**
  Kimchi, Corn, and Scallion
  Fried Rice (leftover)

- **Snack**
  Store-bought hummus
  and veggies

- **Dinner**
  Butternut Squash and Ricotta
  Pizza with Cranberries
  (page 147)

- **Snack**
  "Cheesy" Lemon Pepper
  Popcorn (page 203) (Tip: Make
  extra to enjoy throughout the
  week)

Saturday

- **Breakfast**
  Yogurt with raspberries
  and walnuts

- **Snack**
  Hard-boiled egg and
  bell pepper strips

- **Lunch**
  Butternut Squash and Ricotta
  Pizza with Cranberries (leftover)

- **Snack**
  "Cheesy" Lemon Pepper
  Popcorn (leftover)

- **Dinner**
  Spaghetti with Chickpea-
  Basil Meatballs (page 133)
  (Tip: Make extra meatballs for
  lunch tomorrow)

- **Snack**
  Turmeric Hot Cocoa (page 155)

Sunday

- **Breakfast**
  Avocado Sweet Potato Toast
  with a Fried Egg (page 107)

- **Snack**
  Green tea and pistachios

- **Lunch**
  Chickpea-Basil Meatballs
  (leftover) in a sandwich

- **Snack**
  Store-bought hummus
  and carrots

- **Dinner**
  One-Pot Thai Red Curry
  (page 171) (Tip: Make extra to
  enjoy throughout the week)

- **Snack**
  Mango slices with
  coconut yogurt

SUGGESTED SNACKS + SWEETS

Let's Get Cookin'	Grab 'n' Go
"Cheesy" Lemon Pepper Popcorn (page 203)	Store-bought sea-salt-and-olive-oil popcorn
Turmeric Hot Cocoa (page 155)	Chocolate oat milk
Triple-Berry Lime Smoothie (page 164)	Yogurt with berries
Put-It-on-Everything Dip or Spread (page 204) with veggies	Store-bought hummus with veggies
Peanut Butter Stuffed Dates (page 211)	Dates and peanuts
Green Tea Soft Serve (page 216)	Green tea and pistachios
Fudgy Avocado Walnut Brownies (page 217)	Dark chocolate and walnuts
Pomegranate, Mandarin, and Ginger Smoothie (page 157)	Mandarin and pumpkin seeds
Hummus Deviled Eggs (page 206)	Hard-boiled egg and bell pepper strips
Better-Than-Ever Banana Bread (page 209)	Banana with peanut butter

support immunity

or, "why am I sick all the time?"

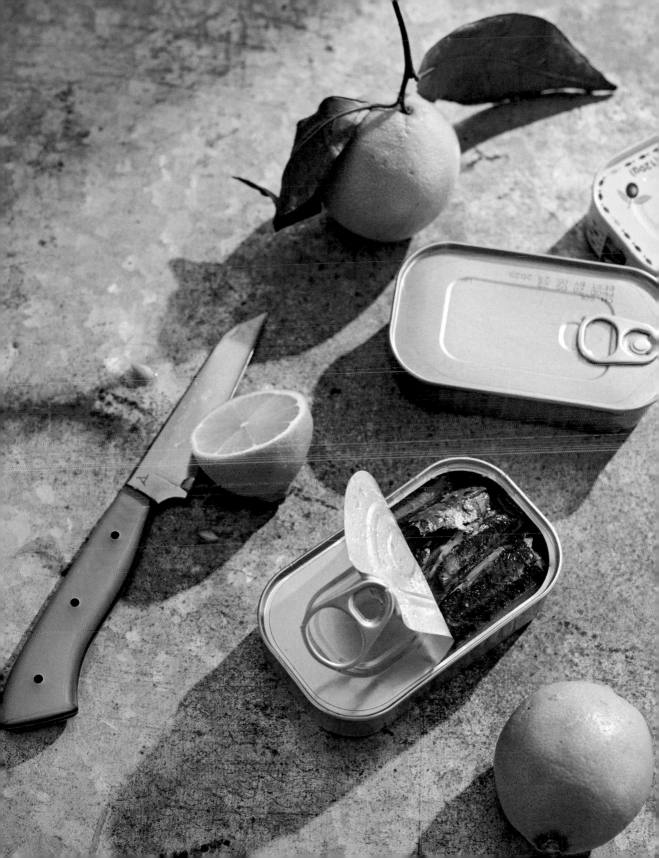

> I have come to believe that caring for myself is not self-indulgent.
> Caring for myself is an act of survival.
> —Audre Lorde

Does "sick and tired" feel like your default mode? You're not alone. It's a vicious cycle: You're sick and worn down and *desperately* need rest, but there's no time for that. You have work. The kids. A social life. And so many items on your to-do list. So you push through, telling yourself to toughen up, get stronger, and quit whining. It's just sniffles.

You chug some orange juice, pop some over-the-counter cold meds, maybe take some zinc or a turmeric shot, and hope for the best. But then your sniffles turn into a cold, which lingers, then becomes a sinus infection or an ear infection or strep throat. Again.

If you feel like you spend most of the winter either actively sick or recovering from yet another bug, it's time to take a new approach to immune health—and that starts with looking at its connection to burnout and to stress. Chronic stress and burnout can take a toll on your immune system. It's hard for your body to fight back against germs when you're overworked and under-rested. Think of your health like you do your attention span. On a good day—when you're well-rested, you've had just enough (but not too much) coffee, and you're feeling your best—you can multitask. You're able to check your email on the treadmill, help your son with his multiplication tables while you cook dinner, or take a work call on your commute home. But when

something goes awry—the incline suddenly increases, the pasta water boils over, or the car in front of you slams on the brakes—you can't divide your attention evenly.

The same thing happens in your body. Your systems and organs are programmed to keep things running smoothly on their own. Every day, each system chugs along, taking its usual amount of effort and energy. Your heart beats. You're breathing steadily. Your temperature and fluid levels are normal. And you don't have to think about any of it. This balance is known as homeostasis. In a perfect world, we all would be healthy and balanced day in and day out. But in real life, stuff happens—like stress.

Stress is a Bravo reality star, demanding attention at any cost. But when it does, your body doesn't magically have more energy to devote to stress. Nope, your bodily functions and systems have to give up some of their portion. Stress shortchanges your immune system, leaving you more vulnerable to illness—and in turn, more stressed.

What is the immune system and how does it work?

At the start of the novel coronavirus pandemic, it became evident how little most of us know about our immune health. We all wanted to learn what we could do to "boost" our immune system—Google Trends showed quite the *boost* in searches for "how to boost your immune system with food," "best vitamin to boost immune system," and more.

That's not how the immune system works—but how are we supposed to know that? Unlike the circulatory system or reproductive system, the immune system doesn't have well-known organs or even any clearly defined roles. "Keeps you healthy" is kinda vague. What does that mean?

Your immune system is a complicated, vast, and widespread network that functions around the clock to prevent or limit infections from head to toe. It works from the inside out and the outside in, and it impacts every other system, organ, and tissue in your body.

Immune cells and tissues are responsible for:

- Cell and tissue repair and replenishment

- Microbiome support and maintenance, in your gut and other mucosal tissues

- Natural detox—like disposing of cells that have reached the end of their life cycle and what's left behind by bodily processes

- Fighting off microbes, pathogens, and other interlopers

Think of your body as a business and the organs, tissues, and cells of your immune system as your employees. Their role? Keeping everything orderly, efficient, and safe every day, every season, and every year. Your immune system has certain tasks that it checks off on a regular basis and others that are done only as needed.

Together your cells, tissues, and organs offer up two types of immunity:

1. **Innate immunity** is built-in and primitive. Your skin, white blood cells, and mucosal linings are your first line of defense to fighting off pathogens and potential infections.

2. **Adaptive immunity** is the backup plan, sort of like the National Guard for your immune system. This part of your immune system steps in when an invader has breached the perimeter, so to speak—that cold virus made it inside or a cut on your finger wasn't cleaned properly.

This duo works together to help prevent you from getting sick—and aid in recovery when you inevitably do.

How to Show Your Immune System Some TLC

Some people "never get sick"—call it luck, fate, or good genes. They won the lottery. As for the rest of us, we can keep slowly and steadily socking away "immunity dividends," letting it build interest, and seeing the benefits over time. Start with these simple tips to invest in your immune system.

1. **Keep active.** Physical activity is good for you, period. When it comes to immune health, exercise stimulates certain aspects of your innate immune system, which improves your body's ability to recognize foreign pathogens over time—and may decrease overall inflammation, too. Every time you exercise, you could also be flushing out your lungs and airways and positively changing your white blood cells and antibodies.

2. **Prioritize sleep.** According to a poll by the National Sleep Foundation, 63 percent of Americans aren't getting enough rest. When you are sleep-deprived, your body is at a higher risk for illness. While everyone is different, aim for seven to nine hours of sleep a night. If you're not getting that much, move up your bedtime by fifteen minutes at a time until you are.

3. **Manage your stress.** Easier said than done, I know. But you have to keep stress in check if you want to stay healthy. Chronic stress takes a toll on the immune system. The link between stress and immune health is undeniable! Find what works for you—and make time for it. Whether it's meditation, a nature walk, or an Epsom salt bath, stress reduction strategies can give your mind a break.

4. **Stay hydrated.** There's a meme that perfectly illustrates why water is so important to good health: *The human body is 90 percent water, so we're basically just cucumbers with anxiety.* Drinking water is one of the best things you can do to keep healthy.

5. **Work on your anger.** Anger is an emotion that many women struggle with—we're taught from a young age that it's not a feeling we should experience or share. However, anger is natural, just like sadness or joy. It can take a toll on your immunity, though. Harvard researchers found that even thinking about a time when you were peeved can cause levels of an immunoprotective antibody (one that's your body's first line of defense) to dip for six hours!

6. **Pile on the produce.** A plant-powered diet— like the recipes and meal plans shared in this book—is good for every aspect of your health, including your immunity. You'll get to know the specific nutrients that impact immune health later on, but all fruits and vegetables are good for your immune system.

What burnout does to your immune system

Let's use tech as an analogy: You can have the latest computer, with the biggest hard drive. But if you don't charge or update that computer regularly, it starts to slow down, freeze, and sometimes stops working entirely. The same goes for your body. Being stressed is like spilling coffee on your keyboard over and over. It's like never deleting a file or installing an update. Burnout is when you have no space left on your hard drive and can't save the important project. It's when the motherboard finally shorts out after one too many spills.

If your body is spending energy to deal with stress, that keeps it from doing its routine immune tasks. As your stress worsens and you spiral toward burnout, your immune system gets less and less of the attention and energy it deserves. When we experience a catastrophe or trauma, its impact goes beyond our emotional well-being to interfere with our immune function.

That can look like:

- A reduced ability to defend against germs and other invaders

- Elevated blood pressure and increased heart rates

- Digestive upset, which interferes with the microbiome's immune functions

- Suppressed immune function due to higher cortisol levels

- Higher inflammation levels

- More unhealthy habits (drinking, smoking, skipping sleep, eating junk food, and so on) that further erode the immune system's efficiency

- Immune cells that are so exhausted they forget what they're supposed to do and engage in "friendly fire" against your body

Lisa experienced the stress-immune connection firsthand when she was in the middle of her own burnout. As a health care worker who's a self-described (now recovering) "type A perfectionist," she "worked her butt off" to get through undergrad, graduate school, and her clinical fellowship. She was driven and eager—and healthy. It wasn't until she moved across the country, started her dream job, and discovered that the work environment was toxic and unsustainable that she started to lose steam.

From day one, she knew the work would be hard. She was using her health degrees in a corporate environment, one that was cutthroat and moved at breakneck speed. Lisa wasn't afraid—she had worked two part-time jobs to put herself through school (and attended full-time). This was different, though. "It was mean," she says, "from the top down. I was always afraid of making a mistake and of being publicly called out. I wasn't built for that type of place. It got to me."

At first, she thought she needed to toughen up, but then she started getting sick all the time. She caught every bug that came through the office, all year long. Lisa had moved from a snowy, gray northeastern city to sunny California. Back home, she had worked in a huge hospital, where she was exposed to patients day in and day out. Yet she had rarely fallen ill. Now, although she was drinking "more green juice than ever before," she was sick all the time—not just with the sniffles or mild colds, but with strep throat. Like clockwork, every couple of months, she felt that familiar pain and sickness: a throat so red and swollen she could barely swallow, a fever that lasted for days, and a bone-weary fatigue that wouldn't end.

Eventually, Lisa had to have her tonsils removed in her early thirties. Her doctor suggested her health problems could be stress related and warned her she'd be down and out for a couple of weeks. She thought she'd be back in the office after a weekend of rest.

Soon she realized: Her life circled around work, and she had no outlet. Getting sick was her body's cry for help, for balance. When she didn't listen, it screamed louder, until finally she listened—and started her path to healing from burnout.

How inflammation fuels the fire of burnout

Inflammation is your body's way of protecting itself against infection. A fever when you have a cold, heat and swelling when a cut gets infected, pain when you twist your ankle—these are ways your body fights back when you get injured or infected. Your immune system is trained to send specialized cells to deal with any potential issue. While the symptoms of inflammation—pain,

warmth, swelling, and redness—aren't comfortable, they're natural and normal. You have to experience them to some extent in order to heal.

Acute or short-term inflammation, like acute or short-term stress, is designed to help you survive. But, as with stress, chronic inflammation can be problematic. Acute stress is when you use the parking brake to keep your car from sliding down a hill. Chronic stress is when that parking brake gets stuck and you're going down the highway at full speed, sparks flying and car parts grinding.

Inflammation is much the same. To continue our car analogy, acute inflammation is the heat and sparks required to get your car running and keep it going. Chronic inflammation is when your engine starts overheating and melting down because it can't properly manage all the different processes that are happening.

Food also plays a role. Your body is like the fastest, sleekest sports car—so when you give it basic gas, it won't run optimally and could eventually break down. That's why you end up feeling run-down and gross when you feed yourself a steady diet of junk (think: fast food and fried foods, sugary drinks and candy, too much wine or cocktails, etc.).

In your body, inflammation escalates from a little extra warmth to a five-alarm blaze when it becomes chronic. Instead of promoting healing, the inflammation starts to break down your tissues and interfere with your immune function.

When your stress levels are manageable, your body has the energy to devote to regulating inflammation. But when stress is so overwhelming that it distracts you, your immune response to cortisol dulls, letting inflammation add up. By managing your stress, you ensure that the batteries are always charged in your smoke alarms.

After her tonsillectomy and subsequent wake-up call, Lisa found healthy outlets for her stress—like working out, talking to her inner circle, and therapy—which gave her immune system a chance to recover and replenish itself. These days, with much less stress and inflammation, she's catching far fewer colds.

Feeding a healthy immune system

Feed a cold, starve a fever? Not so fast. That adage dates back to 1574—and we've learned a thing or two about immunity since the sixteenth century. Burnout makes you feel dried out and worn down, and that includes your immune system. Thankfully, the newer adage *you are what you eat* is a little more true. No single food will miraculously cure you, nor is any one food going to destroy your immune system (unless you're severely allergic).

That said, certain foods offer more support and benefits for your immune system than others. And deficiencies in specific essential nutrients can suppress immunity. As you learned in chapter 2, whole, unprocessed foods that are as close to their natural state as possible form the basis of your burnout recovery meal plan. Many of those same foods can show your immune system some love.

Inflammatory Foods to Limit

- **Added Sugar:** candy, cookies and cakes, added sugars in foods, and sweetened beverages can wreak havoc on your blood sugar, mood, and immune health.

- **Alcohol:** the occasional glass of wine or cocktail is fine, but alcohol has no nutritional value and can impact sleep, immune pathways, and more.

- **Fried foods and trans fats:** these negatively impact your health, including your microbiome.

- **Salt:** while you need some sodium in your diet, too much added salt can impair your immune function and raise your blood pressure.

While this list is important to be aware of, as with all things, healthy eating is about balance. An *obsession* with "clean eating" is not only unnecessary, it will stress you out! And stress is far worse on your immune system than those occasional fried meals or margaritas. It's much healthier to put your energy into choosing foods that make you feel good, rather than avoiding foods or labeling them as "bad" or off-limits, and this book has lots of information on foods to make you feel good!

25 top immunity-supporting foods to include on your grocery list

 Almonds
vitamin E for immune function and antioxidant support, protein for healing and recovery, fiber for immune support

 Broccoli
vitamin C to stimulate antibody production, fiber for immune support

 Cabbage
amino acid glutamine to fuel immune cells, vitamin C to stimulate antibody production, fiber for immune support

 Carrots
vitamin A to regulate immune system and keep skin and mucosal linings healthy, fiber for immune support

 Cayenne pepper
capsaicin to reduce inflammation for immune support

 Cinnamon
antiviral, antibacterial, and antifungal properties to support immune health, polyphenol antioxidants to reduce oxidative stress

 Flaxseeds
fiber for immune support, copper for red blood cell production, protein for healing and recovery

 Ginger
anti-inflammatory and antioxidant properties to support immunity

 Grapefruit
vitamin C to stimulate antibody production, lycopene for antioxidant support (in pink grapefruit), fiber for immune support

 Grapes
polyphenols for immune support, vitamin K for immune and inflammatory responses

 Kale
folate for immune response, vitamin C to stimulate antibody production, vitamin A to regulate immune system and keep skin and mucosal linings healthy, fiber for immune support

 Kefir
probiotics for a healthy gut immune response, vitamin B_{12} for red blood cell production, protein for healing and recovery, vitamin D for immune response

 Miso
probiotics for a healthy gut immune response

Mushrooms

beta-glucans for immune health, copper for red blood cell production, vitamin D to help regulate both innate and adaptive immune function

Pomegranates

vitamin C to stimulate antibody production, flavonoids for immune support, fiber for immune support

Quinoa

fiber for immune support, protein for healing and recovery, folate for immune response, copper for red blood cell production, zinc for immune support and healing

Red bell peppers

vitamin C to stimulate antibody production, vitamin A to regulate immune system and keep skin and mucosal linings healthy, fiber for immune support

Sardines

DHA and EPA omega-3 fats to reduce inflammation and support immune function, protein for healing and recovery, vitamin D for immune response

Shellfish

zinc for immune support and healing, vitamin B_{12} for red blood cell production, protein for healing and recovery

Sweet potato

vitamin A to regulate immune system and keep skin and mucosal linings healthy, fiber for immune support

Tea

polyphenols for antioxidant support and immune response, L-theanine for immune support

Tomatoes

lycopene for antioxidant support, vitamin C to stimulate antibody production, vitamin A for immune function, fiber for immune support

Turmeric

curcumin for antioxidant support and a healthy inflammatory response

Water

hydration for elimination of toxins and other bacteria

Watermelon

vitamin C to stimulate antibody production, lycopene for antioxidant support, vitamin A for immune function

While this cheat sheet can help you quickly choose foods to aid your immunity, see pages 223–31 for a more comprehensive list to help guide your immune-supporting food choices.

1-week immunity-supporting meal plan

This weeklong meal plan is designed to fit into your busy, active life. Use it as written, or take any of the shortcuts I share throughout. The main goal: Chip away at your burnout "debt" while supporting your immune system—not adding to your stress levels! For nights when you're too run-down to cook, swap a dinner recipe for one of the twenty nearly no-cook dinner ideas on pages 38–39. This is a perfect meal plan to reach for during cold and flu season, or any time you start to feel like you're catching a bug.

Monday

- **Breakfast**
  Yogurt with berries

- **Snack**
  Avocado slices on whole-grain crackers

- **Lunch**
  Leafy green salad with tuna

- **Snack**
  Store-bought sea-salt-and-olive-oil popcorn

- **Dinner**
  Garlic, Lentil, and Carrot Soup (page 173) with rustic whole-grain bread

- **Snack**
  Dark chocolate and walnuts

- **Note**
  Make the Apple Citrus Bircher Bowl (page 111) for breakfast tomorrow and extra for the week

Tuesday

- **Breakfast**
  Apple Citrus Bircher Bowl (premade)

- **Snack**
  Hard-boiled egg and bell pepper strips

- **Lunch**
  Garlic, Lentil, and Carrot Soup (leftover)

- **Snack**
  Grapes and cheese

- **Dinner**
  Poblano and Portobello Tacos (page 125)

- **Snack**
  Sleepy Almond Chamomile Cookies (page 218)

- **Note**
  Freeze banana for smoothie tomorrow morning

Wednesday

- **Breakfast**
  Pomegranate, Mandarin, and Ginger Smoothie (page 157)

- **Snack**
  Carrots and peanut butter

- **Lunch**
  Poblano and Portobello Taco filling (leftover) over a green salad

- **Snack**
  Apple Citrus Bircher Bowl (leftover)

- **Dinner**
  Cashew Chinese Salad with Miso Mustard Dressing (page 183) and brown rice (Tip: Pack extra dressing and salad separately for lunch the next day)

- **Snack**
  100% frozen fruit bar

Thursday

Breakfast
Sprouted whole-grain avocado toast

Snack
Apple and cheese

Lunch
Cashew Chinese Salad with Miso Mustard Dressing (leftover)

Snack
Peanut Butter Stuffed Dates (page 211)

Dinner
Lemony Farro and Lentil Bowls with Shrimp and Grapes (page 150)

Snack
Sleepy Almond Chamomile Cookie (leftover)

Friday

Breakfast
Oatmeal with strawberries and cinnamon

Snack
Hummus and veggies

Lunch
Lemony Farro and Lentil Bowls with Shrimp and Grapes (leftover)

Snack
Hard-boiled egg and bell pepper strips

Dinner
Shiitake and Herb Broth in a Hurry (page 167) with brown rice ramen noodles

Snack
Golden Carrot Spice Muffins (page 116)

Saturday

Breakfast
Golden Carrot Spice Muffin (leftover)

Snack
Kefir and a mandarin

Lunch
Plant-based burger

Snack
Watermelon Cucumber Juice (page 163) and pistachios

Dinner
Cabbage, Mushroom, and Snow Pea Stir-Fry (page 128)

Snack
Mango slices with coconut yogurt

Sunday

Breakfast
Smashed Chickpea Artichoke Scramble with Sun-Dried Tomatoes (page 114)

Snack
Watermelon and pistachios

Lunch
Cabbage, Mushroom, and Snow Pea Stir-Fry (leftover)

Snack
Golden Carrot Spice Muffin (leftover)

Dinner
Sweet Potato, Tomato, and Turmeric Soup (page 168) with rustic whole-grain bread (Tip: Make extra to enjoy throughout the coming week, or freeze for the coming months)

Snack
Sleepy Almond Chamomile Cookie (leftover)

SUGGESTED SNACKS + SWEETS

Let's Get Cookin'	Grab 'n' Go
Pomegranate, Mandarin, and Ginger Smoothie (page 157)	Kefir and a mandarin
Peanut Butter Stuffed Dates (page 211)	Dates and peanuts
Turmeric Hot Cocoa (page 155)	Chocolate oat milk
Watermelon Cucumber Juice (page 163) and pistachios	Watermelon and pistachios
"Cheesy" Lemon Pepper Popcorn (page 203)	Store-bought sea-salt-and-olive-oil popcorn
Sleepy Almond Chamomile Cookies (page 218)	Chamomile tea and almonds
Golden Carrot Spice Muffins (page 116)	Carrots and peanut butter
Put-It-on-Everything Dip or Spread (page 204) with veggies	Store-bought hummus and veggies
Hummus Deviled Eggs (page 206)	Hard-boiled egg and bell pepper strips

enhance focus

for when you've said "hmm?" way too many times in a row

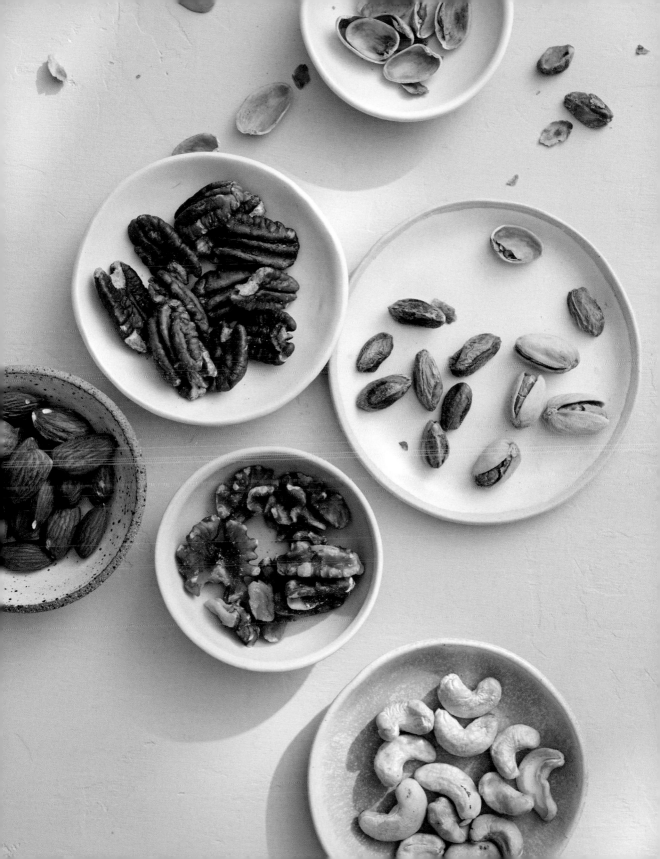

> I've got it all together . . .
> I just forgot where I put it.
> —Anonymous

Much like energy or good hair days, focus can feel out of reach no matter what you do. Sometimes you know why you can't concentrate (a breakup, grief, postpartum hormones, parenting, and working during a pandemic) and other times you do everything "right" and still feel pulled in a million different directions.

A lack of focus and mental clarity were early signs that something was off for me, and they're still reminders that I'm pushing too hard and need a break. I might lose my phone for the third time in a week. Or I'll find a can of chickpeas in the fridge. Sometimes I'll even run the coffee maker without adding water (facepalm!). Can you relate?

A common side effect of burnout, mental fatigue or "brain fog" manifests as sudden mental confusion, inability to focus, and poor memory. Mental fatigue can hamper your clarity to varying degrees, and it's always a red flag. The brain fog that comes with burnout can be terrifying. It goes beyond the usual forgetfulness that happens when you go into a room and can't remember why. (That's called the *doorway effect*, and it's nothing to worry about.) This burnout-induced haze might have you googling the symptoms for early-onset dementia or scouring your family history for Alzheimer's. It's not funny—and it's a common symptom of burnout.

Jacqueline is a born creative whose photography has been featured in books. She's known for intricately styled food photos. And yet, at the height of her burnout, she found herself unable to concentrate long enough to make herself lunch. Even going to the post office felt like too much to handle. While she knew that stress was the culprit, feeling like your brain isn't working right is scary when you're in your thirties, especially for a single woman and entrepreneur.

Thankfully for Jacqueline—and for you—the cognitive decline you can experience during burnout isn't permanent. In this chapter, you'll learn why stress can do this (hint: it's a take-no-prisoners attention fiend, remember?) and what you can do to keep your brain healthy now and as you age. Plus, you'll get a whole week of brain-food meals, snacks, and recipes.

Burnout and the brain

If you looked at a brain scan of a person who has lived through trauma next to the scan of someone dealing with burnout, it might be hard to tell who's who, since burnout can alter a person's brain similarly to emotional trauma. A 2014 research review concluded that burnout impacts cognitive function, causing symptoms ranging from a lack of creativity and struggles with solving problems to memory issues and attention lapses.

This isn't just zoning out during the middle of your sixth Zoom meeting of the day or forgetting the point you were trying to make during a heated discussion with your tween. Burnout can make you feel like a thick fog has descended upon your brain. It makes you feel dull, spacey, or forgetful. It might even make you question whether you're losing your mind.

So what can you do to heal and clear the cobwebs? A 2012 review of burnout in mental health services offers some helpful suggestions. Even though these strategies were targeted for workplace programming, I found them inspiring for my personal life— and believe they can apply to anyone feeling overwhelmed by stress, at home or at work.

Objective	How to Make It Happen
Find more ways to cope with stress.	Keep a list of things to do when you start to feel overwhelmed. Then do one of them. That might mean sitting in your parked car with the radio cranked, singing at the top of your lungs. It could be walking to get a cold brew when you feel like rolling your eyes at coworkers. Or maybe you go for a run and leave your partner to handle dinner.
Tap your social networks for help.	Asking for help is tough, but nothing will change if nothing changes. Talk to your boss, partner, friends, or other parents in your circle. Find ways to share the burden and divide up the work. Is your workload unrealistic? Could you ask someone to cohost your friend's surprise party with you? Can your in-laws help with school pickup one afternoon a week?
Reclaim your intrinsic motivation.	Think about what motivates (or motivated) you. How can you find it again? This might take some time, but reminding yourself why you do what you do—for your business, your friends, your kids, or your sweetheart—can make those days when you "can't even" feel more manageable. When motivation comes from within versus from external influences, it's more likely to stick.
Practice gratitude.	Too often, women are pressured to perform gratitude and sugarcoat our problems. That doesn't help alleviate stress—and you don't need to apologize for feeling strife, even if others around you have harder lives. Instead, use gratitude as a way to find the light during darker times. At the end of each day, write down what you're grateful for—and go ahead and jot down what you're resenting, too.

Objective	How to Make It Happen
Find more meaning.	Burnout has a way of stealing your worth and making you feel not just like an imposter, but like an actor or a mime. When you reconnect with why you made your life choices in the first place, getting through the rough patches feels possible. If you're a person of faith, reconnect to that side of you. If not, think about what refills your cup. Is it watching your little one learn something new? Helping a customer overcome a problem? The look on your partner's face when they come home and see you? For the days that feel heavy, keep a reminder of your "why" nearby—a photo of friends or family, a note from that customer, or a cherished token from your love.
Avoid numbing out.	That extra glass of wine. Bingeing an entire series on Netflix. A pint of cookie dough ice cream. Back-to-back spin classes. Working late (again). Scrolling Instagram. We all have ways to dull the pain and tune out our feelings. But that'll only keep you in burnout longer. Instead, figure out how you numb out—and do those things less often. Refer back to the top of the list and slowly start to work in healthier ways to cope with stress.
Unload some of your work.	The world will not end if you don't do everything yourself. Let go of the mommy martyr or girl boss or Wonder Woman ideal and take some help. Maybe you use a meal kit service instead of cooking every dinner from scratch. Or you have the kids load the dishwasher, even if they don't do it the way you showed them. Perhaps you even tell your manager no or let your coworker lead this project.
Assign chores and tasks.	Asking for help is hard because it usually makes work for you up front. Instead of waiting until you're stressed and tired to ask for things one at a time, look for tasks and responsibilities to take off your plate permanently. When it's always your husband's job to clean the litter box, asking him to do it won't take up space or require your emotional labor. When your sitter always helps the kids clean their room or folds laundry, you don't have to remember to ask about it. Families are teams, and teams help each other—so find ways to have everyone do their part!

Different types and degrees of mental exhaustion

Mental exhaustion is different from physical exhaustion. The latter is easier to identify and reverse, at least in the short term. Mental exhaustion is trickier, more complex. Thanks to research, we know there are two types: 1) impaired performance during tasks, and 2) slowed reaction times and feeling sleepy. These two types of fatigue change the brain in different ways because they impact different areas of the brain.

You're more likely to feel mentally wiped out in situations that demand more of your attention and focus—like work meetings or crowded social settings. But exhaustion can also show up when you're alone: you can't focus when you try to read a book in bed, or you lose your place when trying to recount a story to your spouse. Symptoms of mental fatigue and cognitive signs of burnout can impact your emotional, behavioral, and physical health and well-being. It's a reminder that burnout isn't all in your head—it affects your entire life.

We often feel unfocused and distracted even when we're not completely burned out. When you're ready to gnaw off your own arm right before lunch and your blood sugar is low, can you give your boss a clear answer? What about when you've been up all night with a sick toddler? How about when you're ill, depressed, or anxious? It comes down to resource management. Those other issues are more important, so they're taking more of the energy your body has to spare today. And of course, you can't forget about stress. When you're in fight-or-flight mode, it's like having a fire alarm blaring inside your body. Good luck focusing on anything with that in the background!

A Lack of Focus Could Be ADHD

If you feel like focus has been an issue since long before you felt burnout, it could be attention-deficit/hyperactivity disorder (ADHD), a treatable condition that's often overlooked or misdiagnosed in women. Instead, we're told it's our hormones, or stress. Oftentimes we're told it's burnout.

Symptoms of ADHD vary—and they're much different in children. In adults, ADHD can look like burnout, with signs including:

- A short fuse or mood swings
- Clutter and disorganization
- Struggles to manage a household, finances, or work
- Inability to handle stress
- Multitasking and time management problems

  Women may also experience:

- Depression and/or anxiety
- Exhaustion
- Inability to focus on details
- Problems with sleeping
- Self-esteem issues

If your inability to focus or complete tasks starts to get in the way of your work, parenting, relationships, or everyday life, you might want to talk to your doctor about it.

Work smarter, not longer

How many hours do you work each week? What about running your household and parenting? Do you feel like you're productive the entire time? If you're working more than forty hours a week, that might be contributing to both your burnout and your mental fatigue. According to a groundbreaking study from the UK, people who worked more than fifty-five hours a week didn't perform as well on vocabulary tests and other cognitive assessments as those who worked forty hours or fewer. And during a follow-up study a few years later, long work hours predictably led to a decline in performance on reasoning tests. A report from the CDC on overtime and the impact of working long shifts further endorses the idea of working smarter, not longer:

- Working overtime was linked to overall poor health.

- During a twelve-hour shift, most people reported symptoms like decreased alertness, impaired cognition, fatigue, and reduced vigilance starting around the ninth hour.

- Working twelve-hour-plus shifts *and* more than forty hours a week was linked to a slower work pace, more health issues, and poorer performance.

- Injuries, performance, health behaviors, and morale were all impacted by longer workdays.

Working basically twenty-four/seven for years was how Jacqueline burned out. "I'd been working sixty-hour weeks for probably fifteen years, often working closer to eighty hours a week with little social life or self-care time and eating most meals at my desk."

An emotional shutdown and existential crisis helped her see she needed to scale back. A lack of energy and focus were her biggest symptoms, but she also dealt with muscle weakness, sore joints, dizziness, nausea, trouble sleeping at night, excessive daytime sleepiness, weight gain, inflammation, overactive bladder, hair loss, and kaleidoscopic vision at times.

Ultimately, she closed three of her four businesses—"a scary step," she admits. "I wasn't sure I could earn the amount of money I needed to survive, but it turns out I was able to devote the right amount of time to get the business to grow."

Not only is Jacqueline doing fine financially, but she's also able to focus on work when she's working and still be present in her social life (she has one now!) "Before, it was really easy to grab my attention and pull me in a direction without me even considering if it was something worth my time and energy," confesses Jacqueline. "Now I look at my own needs first, then at the validity of the request. Am I the best person to solve this problem? Is this request a need or a want? What are the pros and cons of saying yes or no?"

This is a lesson Tamika learned, too. "You're more than your job," she says. "Rather than striving to be content, everybody wants us to be this best version. But that ends up being unattainable. I lived my life putting in full effort, full dedication—giving 120 percent every day. I didn't do anything half-assed. And then it caught up with me. Now I'm okay doing less and giving less—but I'm not any less of a person. I learned where I could cut corners. As a full-time working mother, you have to cut corners. And that's okay."

Emotional labor and decision fatigue

If you're a woman with a family, chances are you carry out most of the emotional labor in your household. As such, you're responsible for more of the decisions that keep everyone else healthy and happy. You and only you decide things like which dress your daughter will wear for school pictures, which photo package you'll buy, whether you'll put her hair in braids or leave it down, and, later, which family members to send photos (and you'll likely have to remember to go to the post office, too).

It's estimated that adults make 35,000 decisions a day. I'd wager that most women make at least half of those for other people. Over time, we start to experience decision fatigue. This happens when we're low on energy and motivation, and our stress is high. We're faced with a choice—but also have an empty tank.

Decision fatigue is why you might cave and let your teen stay out until midnight even though you regret it as soon as they leave home. It's why you add on the large order of fries in the drive-through when you intended to pick up a salad after a long shift. And decision fatigue is what compels you to snap at your boyfriend, "I don't care, just pick one," after he asks you what restaurant you want to go to.

So what can you do about it? Eliminate the need to make decisions. Put things on autopilot. Schedule subscriptions or autorenewals. Delegate tasks to someone else. And consider being more like Matilda Kahl.

Kahl, a New York art director, was tired of running late after struggling to pick out the perfect outfit. She bought fifteen identical white shirts and six pairs of the same black pants—and she has worn them for three years and counting. Men, including my husband most days, do this all the time. (He has a shelf of twenty black T-shirts and they're pretty much the only shirts he wears). And no one notices. It's a brilliant idea!

Identify where you waste time and mental energy making decisions every day, then stop making them. You might:

- Eat the same breakfast every single day or pack the same lunch instead of stressing about what to make as you're running out the door.

- Run the same three-mile loop Monday, Wednesday, and Friday, so you'll never end up losing track of time.

- Buy your son the same brand and color of sneakers every three months when he inevitably outgrows them.

- Set reminders in your calendar to alert you two weeks before events like Aunt Sarah's birthday, so you don't forget to buy cards. (And buy those in bulk, so you don't have to pick one out every time.)

Automating choices like these can help you retain more of your self-control, which is a limited resource and gets depleted each time you have to pause and ponder a decision.

The Power of Saying No

One of the best habits I developed as I healed from burnout was learning to say no. These days, I remind myself: *If you can't say no, you can't say yes.* Saying no was hard to learn! I'm a pleaser by nature, and I'm driven—I like accomplishing things and crushing goals. But by saying yes to everyone else, I was saying no to me, which left me with less time and energy to give to those I love most.

If you're burned (or burning) out, you can't keep doing what you're doing. You have to free up some time and space—and that means learning to say no. Know this: If you feel like the world expects women to say yes, you're right. Research at Rice University in 2014 confirmed this. As natural caregivers, women are expected to step up and take on extra tasks (administrative duties, party planning, etc.)—and our peers' and managers' impressions of us are affected when we decline the additional work.

Here are a few tips to help you learn to say no.

1. **Start small.** Practice saying no and declining invitations from people you know won't hold it against you. Skip this month's book club, tell your sister you can't help plan Thanksgiving, or let your coworker down gently when they ask you to bring in dessert. As you gain confidence, you'll be able to decline more—and bigger—asks.

2. **Close the window.** How many times have you prefaced your no with "I'd love to, but . . . " or "I wish I could . . . "? Same. That polite intro to your refusal leaves open the window of opportunity. It turns your no into a maybe. Before you say no, take a deep breath and dive in—but leave out the first part. (And don't follow up with "Maybe next time," unless you really mean it.)

3. **Change "can't" to "don't."** Researchers in 2011 found that shifting your response from "I can't . . . " to "I don't . . . " was a more effective way to say no. The latter implies that saying yes would violate your personal rules or habits, while the former feels like that no might be up for debate. So, instead of saying "I can't help with the class Halloween party," you might say, "I don't have the flexibility to leave work during the day."

Boost your cognitive powers to feel more joy and serenity

Brain fog is one of the worst symptoms of burnout, but you can manage it—and eventually reverse it, coming out on the other side as your usual focused and sharp self. Thankfully, there are plenty of wellness solutions to help you boost your cognitive powers, enhance your memory, and maybe even protect your brain as you age.

Here are ten simple ones worth trying.

1. **Don't skip meals.** Your brain needs glucose to function. So when you skip meals or go too long without eating, that fog and fuzziness you feel is your brain begging for fuel. Keep healthy snacks around—a balanced mix of protein, fiber, and fats—to keep your blood-sugar levels steady and ward off hangry-induced distractions.

2. **Make a list.** Make technology your BFF to help you track tasks and lists on the go. If someone asks you for a favor at work or in your personal life, tell them to send you an email so you're less likely to let it slip through the cracks.

3. **Streamline your choices.** Decision fatigue can erode your energy and focus. By reducing the number of choices you have, you reduce the number of decisions you have to make. This also works with finicky toddlers who are embracing their independent streaks but struggle to choose which one toy will come along to the playground.

4. **Focus on one thing.** Multitasking actually impairs productivity, according to the American Psychological Association. Toggling between tasks can cost you 40 percent of your efficiency. Instead, embrace a single-minded approach to work. Do one thing from start to finish, then do another. Turn off notifications, close your web browser, and block out distractions—you may be surprised at how much you can get done this way. And, if you can, group similar activities and tasks together. For me, this might mean doing recipe development on one day, having client and brand meetings the next, and writing my book on another.

5. **Make exercise a priority.** Beyond boosting your mood, the hormones released when you work out can also help your attention and focus. Try making morning workouts part of your routine, so you'll feel fresh and focused earlier in the day—and you won't get behind on work or too distracted to make time for exercise. If you love long and steady workouts, you're in luck: Your endurance exercise offers your brain an extra bonus, thanks to the release of a molecule called irisin that impacts both memory and learning.

6. **Exercise your mind, too.** Your brain looks for shortcuts, often choosing well-worn paths between neurons instead of forging new ones. But when we learn something new that demands our attention, thus creating a new pathway, we help our brain stay sharp and agile. Crosswords are helpful, but they're not enough. Focus on activities that challenge you—like (re)learning geometry alongside your tween or taking up archery. When it comes to brain health, it's use it or lose it as we age!

7. **Put your phone down.** Talk about a familiar pathway. Scrolling is a numbing activity for so many of us. Seeing those likes, new posts, and top headlines gives us a little hit of dopamine, and it distracts us from whatever we should be doing. While social media is a wonderful way to broaden your network, learn about the experiences of others, and stay connected to your people (which can help prevent cognitive decline as you age), it's also distracting. Use the time limits available on your device, and put some rules in place for yourself—as you might for your kids.

8. **Clear your mind.** Ironic as it might seem, clearing your mind might help you focus. Meditation changes your brain patterns—and it also boosts cognitive performance. You don't need to do a silent retreat to benefit from meditation. Download an app on your phone and start with a couple of minutes a day. Instead of thinking of meditation as a way to empty your mind, think of it as clearing the clutter. You stay focused on your breath and the present moment regardless of the thoughts that come to mind or the distractions that pop up. If burnout is impacting your record at work, make time for meditation. A 2019 study found that even twenty minutes of guided meditation could help you reduce the number of mistakes you make!

9. **Breathe through it.** Your brain needs oxygen, which you get less of when you're taking shallow breaths during times of stress. Deep breathing can not only train your brain to stay focused on a task but also help you manage stress (and hopefully avoid brain fog in the first place).

10. **Sleep on it.** Fatigue makes it hard to concentrate, no doubt about it. When you're struggling with burnout or insomnia, sleep may not come easily. In addition to a solid eight hours at night, a nap during the day could help you beat brain fog. Research from 2010 supported short naps (five to fifteen minutes) as a way to temporarily improve performance. The results will last one to three hours, so time your siesta accordingly (early afternoon is best). Don't hit the snooze button, though: the study also found that napping for more than thirty minutes can impair brain function!

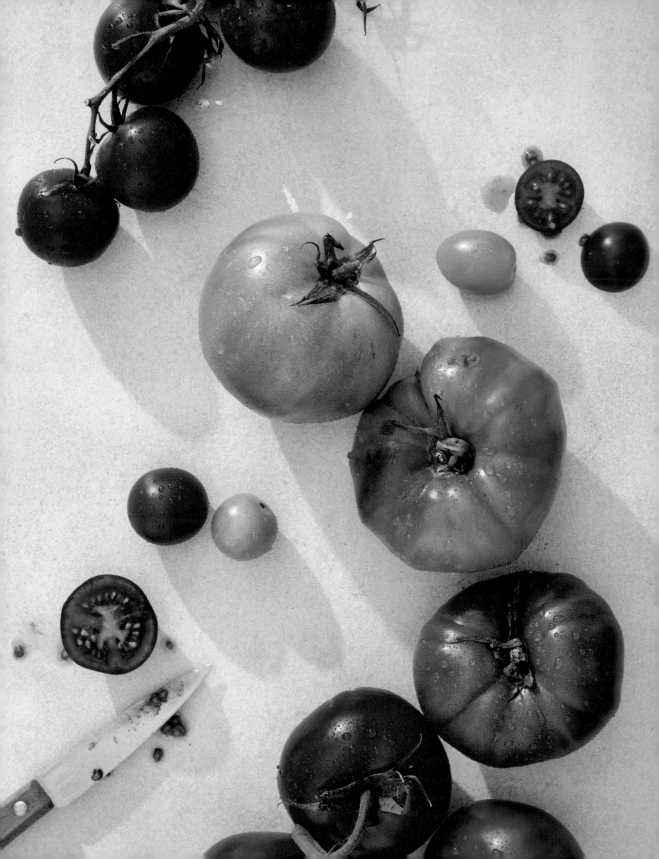

Polyphenols for Brain Health

Polyphenols, found in most fruits and vegetables, are powerful plant-based compounds with antioxidant properties. They are known to influence a number of biological systems relevant to brain health, and are one of the main reasons berries, grapes, and dark chocolate have been shown to promote cognitive health.

Not only can berries—including strawberries, raspberries, blackberries, and blueberries—help improve memory issues as we age, they can also delay cognitive decline, according to research. That's due to their flavonoids (a type of polyphenol antioxidant), which can actually cross the blood-brain barrier to access regions involved in learning and memory.

Grapes are another fruit packed with polyphenols, such as resveratrol, which has been widely studied for its health benefits, including immune function, cancer prevention, and cognition. In a preliminary study conducted at UCLA, researchers found that grapes may support brain health by preserving healthy metabolic activity in areas of the brain where decline is associated with early-stage Alzheimer's.

Dark chocolate also provides flavonoids, which help out with production of neurons, aid in maintaining cerebral blood flow and supply, and support brain function.

The food and brain connection

Back in chapter 3, when we talked about mood, you learned about the gut-brain connection. That same axis impacts focus and cognitive health. Deficiencies of certain essential nutrients can cause cognitive issues, and so can food intolerances. While the jury is still out on whether gut flora is the cause or effect of age-related cognitive issues, we do know there's a connection. We also know that brain health and inflammation are linked, as you read in chapter 4. The concept of "brain food" is real—and we'll learn about foods that impact your brain in this chapter.

The big takeaway is that a diverse diet packed with plants will help you age better. In Canada, researchers studied the diets of nearly 8,600 people who were middle-aged or older. Those who ate more plants (fruits, vegetables, nuts, and pulses) were less likely to demonstrate cognitive decline. The study used a test of verbal fluency, where respondents listed as many words in a category as they could in a certain amount of time. More plants - a bigger vocabulary.

Of course, plants are not the only foods that benefit your brain. Read on to see which ones made my top twenty-five brain foods list.

25 foods to include on your grocery list for better brain function

 Arugula
nitrates to increase blood flow to the brain, vitamin K to regulate calcium for a healthy brain, vitamin A for mental flexibility

 Avocado
healthy fats for brain function and memory, magnesium for healthy cerebral blood flow, vitamin C to protect against dementia, vitamin K to regulate calcium for a healthy brain

 Barley
B vitamins to support neurotransmitter production, fiber for blood sugar stability, iron to support oxygen transport to the brain

 Beans
B vitamins to support neuro-transmitter production, fiber for blood sugar stability, protein for a healthy brain and nervous system

 Beets
complex carbs for brain fuel, fiber for blood sugar stability, nitrates to increase blood flow to the brain

 Blueberries
vitamin C to protect against dementia, flavonoids to improve memory and delay cognitive decline

 Brussels sprouts
vitamin C to protect against dementia, vitamin K to regulate calcium for a healthy brain, vitamin A for mental flexibility

 Butternut squash
carotenoid (beta-carotene) may protect the brain from mental decline, fiber for blood sugar stability, vitamin C to protect against dementia

 Cauliflower
glucosinolates to protect blood vessels from cognitive decline, vitamin C to protect against dementia, vitamin K to regulate calcium for a healthy brain

 Coffee (in moderation)
caffeine for mental clarity, antioxidants to help slow brain aging

 Dark chocolate
polyphenols to support production of neurons for brain function and maintain cerebral blood flow and supply

 Edamame
protein for a healthy brain and nervous system, iron to support oxygen transport to the brain, magnesium for healthy cerebral blood flow, vitamin K to regulate calcium for a healthy brain

 Eggs
vitamin D for cognitive function, protein for a healthy brain and nervous system, carotenoids for focus and mental flexibility, choline to support working memory

Grapes
polyphenols to improve memory and preserve healthy brain function, vitamin K to regulate calcium for a healthy brain

 Greek yogurt
protein for a healthy brain and nervous system, probiotics for mood and cognitive function

 Green tea
polyphenols to protect cells from damage related to oxidative stress, L-theanine for a calm yet alert state, caffeine for mental clarity

 Nutritional yeast
B vitamins to support neurotransmitter production, protein for a healthy brain and nervous system, fiber for blood sugar stability

 Olives and olive oil
healthy fats for brain function and memory, vitamin E to protect brain cells

 Oranges
vitamin C to protect against dementia, flavonoids to improve memory and delay cognitive decline, fiber for blood sugar stability

 Pistachios
protein for a healthy brain and nervous system, fiber for blood sugar stability, antioxidants to help slow brain aging

 Pomegranates
flavonoids to improve memory and delay cognitive decline, vitamin C to protect against dementia, vitamin K to regulate calcium for a healthy brain, fiber for blood sugar stability

 Sunflower seeds
vitamin E to protect brain cells, B vitamins to support neurotransmitter production, magnesium for healthy cerebral blood flow, fiber for blood sugar stability

 Tomatoes
vitamin C to protect against dementia, lycopene to reduce inflammation and neurological stress

 Trout
vitamin D for cognitive function, magnesium for healthy cerebral blood flow, protein for a healthy brain and nervous system, omega-3 fats for brain function and memory

 Walnuts
polyphenols to support memory, protein for a healthy brain and nervous system, fiber for blood sugar stability, magnesium for healthy cerebral blood flow

While this cheat sheet can help you quickly choose foods that support your brain health, see pages 223–31 for a more comprehensive list of foods and nutrients that support focus.

1-week focus-enhancing meal plan

This is the meal plan for the weeks when you need to be on top of your game, mentally, as well as for those weeks when you're experiencing brain fog. Whether you have a big client presentation or simply can't find your keys (again!), this meal plan will fuel your body and brain so that you have the mental stamina and focus you need. "Brain food" doesn't have to be complicated or time-consuming; as with the other weeks, you have the option to take shortcuts, use freezer meals strategically, or swap a dinner recipe for one of the twenty nearly no-cook dinner ideas on pages 38–39.

To limit decision fatigue, this meal plan has you repeat the same breakfast each weekday morning. If you're not a fan of oatmeal, start each day with avocado toast or yogurt and berries. Whatever it is, you'll find relief having one less decision to make when you wake.

Monday

- **Breakfast**
  Oatmeal with nuts and berries

- **Snack**
  Hard-boiled egg and bell pepper strips

- **Lunch**
  Plant-based burger

- **Snack**
  Banana and peanut butter

- **Dinner**
  Broccoli Mandarin Salad with Ginger Scallion Dressing (page 189) and wild rice

- **Snack**
  Pumpkin Spice Almond Butter Balls (page 212)

Tuesday

- **Breakfast**
  Oatmeal with nuts and berries

- **Snack**
  Pumpkin Spice Almond Butter Balls (leftover)

- **Lunch**
  Broccoli Mandarin Salad with Ginger Scallion Dressing and wild rice (leftover)

- **Snack**
  Grapes and cheese

- **Dinner**
  Fettuccine with Tuna, Edamame, and Pistachios (page 138)

- **Snack**
  Triple-Berry Lime Smoothie (page 164)

Wednesday

- **Breakfast**
  Oatmeal with nuts and berries

- **Snack**
  Apple and cheese

- **Lunch**
  Fettuccine with Tuna, Edamame, and Pistachios (leftover)

- **Snack**
  Pumpkin Spice Almond Butter Balls (leftover)

- **Dinner**
  Mediterranean Eggplant Hummus Bowl (page 130) with Fresh Herb Hummus (page 131) (Tip: Make extra Fresh Herb Hummus to enjoy throughout the week)

- **Snack**
  "Cheesy" Lemon Pepper Popcorn (page 203)
  Note: Freeze bananas for soft serve tomorrow

Thursday

● **Breakfast**
Oatmeal with nuts and berries

● **Snack**
Hard-boiled egg with bell pepper strips

● **Lunch**
Fresh Herb Hummus (leftover) in a veggie wrap

● **Snack**
Green Tea Soft Serve (page 216)

● **Dinner**
Ultimate Caprese Salad Flatbread (page 123)

● **Snack**
"Cheesy" Lemon Pepper Popcorn (leftover)

Friday

● **Breakfast**
Oatmeal with nuts and berries

● **Snack**
Fresh Herb Hummus (leftover) and carrots

● **Lunch**
Ultimate Caprese Salad Flatbread (leftover)

● **Snack**
Green Tea Soft Serve (leftover)

● **Dinner**
Cauliflower and Black Bean Chili (page 174)

● **Snack**
Mini Lemon Blueberry Muffins (page 210)

Saturday

● **Breakfast**
Mini Lemon Blueberry Muffins (leftover)

● **Snack**
Green tea and pistachios

● **Lunch**
Cauliflower and Black Bean Chili (leftover)

● **Snack**
Hard-boiled egg and bell pepper strips

● **Dinner**
Simple Salmon Burgers with Grape Salsa (page 144)

● **Snack**
Strawberry Pecan Crisp (page 221)

Sunday

● **Breakfast**
Shaved Asparagus and Potato Frittata (page 108)

● **Snack**
Banana with peanut butter

● **Lunch**
Simple Salmon Burger patty (leftover) over a green salad

● **Snack**
Green Tea Soft Serve (leftover)

● **Dinner**
Miso Soup with Greens and Tofu (page 176) with brown rice noodles (Tip: Make extra to enjoy throughout the coming week, or freeze for the coming months)

● **Snack**
Mini Lemon Blueberry Muffins (leftover)

SUGGESTED SNACKS + SWEETS

Let's Get Cookin'	Grab 'n' Go
Green Tea Soft Serve (page 216)	Green tea and pistachios
Blueberry Cacao Smoothie (page 159)	Dark chocolate and blueberries
Hummus Deviled Eggs (page 206)	Hard-boiled egg and bell pepper strips
Mini Lemon Blueberry Muffins (page 210)	Yogurt with berries
Turmeric Hot Cocoa (page 155)	Chocolate oat milk
"Cheesy" Lemon Pepper Popcorn (page 203)	Store-bought sea-salt-and-olive-oil popcorn
Strawberry Pecan Crisp (page 221)	Strawberries and pecans
Pumpkin Spice Almond Butter Balls (page 212)	Whole-food snack bar
Fresh Herb Hummus (page 131) and veggies	Store-bought hummus and veggies
Five-Ingredient Chocolate Chip–Banana Oat Bites (page 207)	Banana with peanut butter

promote sleep

strategies for shutting off a racing mind

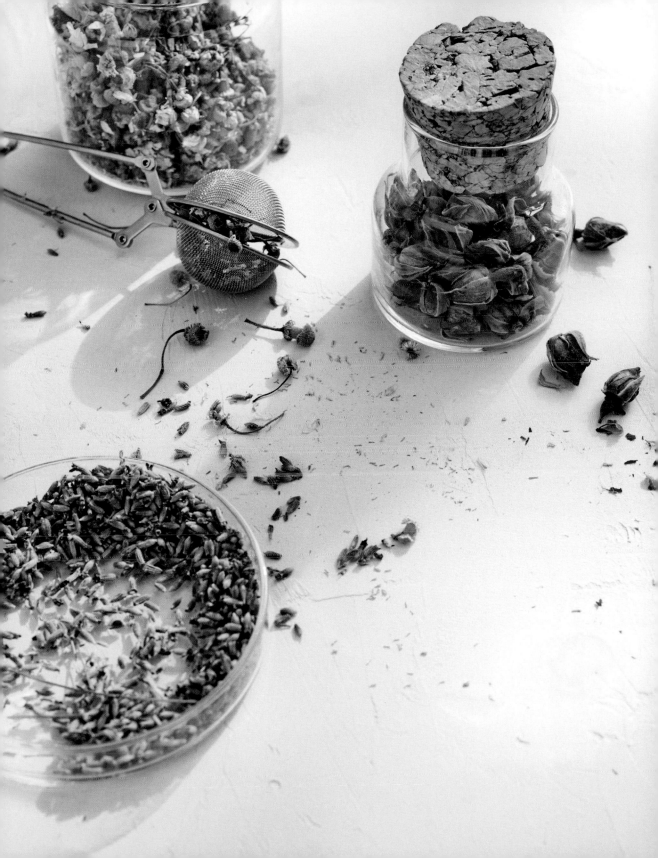

"I can sleep when I'm dead." —Me, age 25

"I'd kill for a good night's sleep." —Me, age 35

—Anonymous

Remember when you could stay up all night—studying, working, drinking, having sex, talking on the phone, or *whatever*—then wake up after a couple of hours of sleep and still look and feel ready to face the day? What I wouldn't give to have that ability back again!

Somewhere around age thirty, that shifted. Sleep suddenly went from optional to mandatory. A good night's sleep, elusive as it is at times, was what I craved most. I'd (reluctantly) get out of bed and immediately count down the hours until I could get right back into bed at night. But despite how much I longed to slide under the covers and drift off, sleep always ended up shoved farther down my list of priorities. (Just one more email to send. Just one more basket of laundry to fold. Just one more episode . . . you get my drift, right?) Even if I did get to bed early, my mind usually raced until the wee hours of the morning.

If you think about sleep the way you used to think about sex, you're not alone. Back in 2017, a survey by the Better Sleep Council found that nearly 80 percent of women craved sleep over sex. Just about 42 percent of men agreed. (More on the complicated connection between sleep and sex later.)

Sleep deprivation is so common among the women I talk to about burnout—especially the mothers. And for women who have kids *and* work, too? Sleep deprivation is the rule, not the exception. It's so commonplace that many women don't even try to fight it. They just give in, doing their best to keep their heads above water.

Mireille spent eighteen months stuck in the "I can't sleep" cycle. With two young kids, a demanding sales job, and a lengthy commute in a country and culture that were new to her, she just kept making excuses. But one sleepless night turned into weeks, months, and then more than a year. Relying on caffeine and sleeping in fits and starts became normal, and she eventually adjusted—or so she thought.

According to the American Academy of Sleep Medicine, the main symptom of sleep deprivation is feeling overly tired during the day. No surprise there. But sleep deprivation can also cause:

- Anxiety or depression

- Distraction and reduced vigilance

- Impaired coordination

- Inability to concentrate

- Increased errors and forgetfulness

- Irritability

- Loss of motivation

- Reduced capacity for decision making

- Reduced energy

- Restlessness

- Slowed reaction times

And that doesn't begin to address the physical side effects. Nothing cures a lack of sleep except sleep—and it must be *good* sleep. A nap can help a little, and so can caffeine for a few hours, but those effects are short-lived and may even cause a rebound effect. Long term, sleep deprivation can lead to major health issues and may affect mortality rates!

Finding a way to prioritize sleep can give you your life back. That's what happened to Mireille and to me. The following questions can help you start to shift awareness to your sleep quality:

- When was the last time you felt truly rested?

- When was the last time you slept through the night and awoke naturally, feeling refreshed?

- What's the first thing you sacrifice when your to-do list overflows?

- How many times in the last week have you wished for more sleep?

- What about the last month or the last year?

- Do you find yourself staring at the ceiling all night?

- Do you wake up when the alarm sounds, only to feel like you just climbed into bed?

- Do you wake up in the middle of the night, unable to fall back to sleep?

- Do you feel stuck in the bad sleep habits you developed during a stressful time—like the big merger at work or when your youngest child was colicky?

- Do you work nights or swing shifts and can't get on a schedule?

You don't have to label or enumerate your sleep issues to start to address them. "I can't sleep" is enough information to get started.

Sleep and Stress and Sex

Can't seem to get in the mood when you're tired? Stress directly interferes with both sleep and sexual desire. Think back to the tiger analogy: If you're outrunning danger, you don't have time to think about jumping into bed to make a baby. When it comes to matters of life and death (which is what your fight-or-flight response may consider your situation to be), your body will choose to focus on preserving the life you have, not creating a new one.

When you're too stressed to sleep, your hormones change, telling your body to dial down sex hormones like estrogen and testosterone so it can boost cortisol production instead. Shifting hormones during and after pregnancy and menopause may be partly to blame, but so are the demands of simply being alive and being a woman. (See also: emotional labor.)

A 2019 study of postmenopausal women found that having "highly stress-reactive sleep systems"—aka being unable to sleep due to a racing mind, anxious thoughts, and so on—is connected to sexual dissatisfaction. Women who can't sleep report changes in libido, challenges achieving orgasm, and reduced desire, as well as issues like pain with intercourse or vaginal dryness. The connection between sleep and sex is so strong that researchers have floated the idea that sleep disorders could be risk factors for sexual dysfunction.

And the self-reported Women's Health Initiative observational study of over 93,000 women ages fifty to seventy-nine supports the idea that, while sleep isn't *better than* sex, it's a key ingredient for *better sex*. Women who clocked less than seven hours of shut-eye a night had sex less often—and were less sexually satisfied—than women who slept more.

Further research into women of all ages has found that getting more sleep increases arousal, and women in relationships who get an extra hour of sleep are 14 percent more likely to have sex. (Remind your partner of this stat the next time you want to sleep in!)

But if you do find yourself in the mood despite your exhaustion, know this: A solo or partnered romp might help you sleep! Some research, including a 2016 review, found that sex before bed could help reduce stress temporarily—and might help women dealing with insomnia fall asleep and stay asleep.

Relationship between burnout, stress, and insomnia

The sleep and stress/burnout relationship reminds me of my daughter's toddler years, when she was overtired but refused to nap and fought bedtime. When I was burning out, insomnia made me feel more like a cranky toddler than like myself. Just making it through the day without wanting to break down felt like a challenge.

I've yet to meet a woman in burnout who has a healthy sleep schedule. The two simply cannot coexist. When you're burned out you can't sleep, and not being able to sleep can cause you to burn out. Insomnia, the official name for the condition of not being able to fall asleep and/or stay asleep, is closely associated with burnout. There is hope, though. The best time to prioritize your sleep is before you burn out, but if you're already in burnout (or careening downhill toward it), focusing on sleep may help.

It's pretty much impossible to be exhausted and feel great at the same time. And the reality is, most of us are tired all too often. According to a 2020 poll by the National Sleep Foundation, 55 percent of Americans say they aren't sleeping well enough (only 44 percent blame a lack of time to sleep). And what do we do about it? Despite reporting headaches, feeling "unwell," and being more irritable, six in ten of us try to "shake it off." Clearly we need a better plan. I hope this chapter serves that purpose for you.

Why sleep is so important

When you don't get enough sleep, your body might pretend like it's business as usual, but behind the scenes, it's panicking: Sleep is the time when your brain sorts through and organizes all the memories and new information you learned during the day. It's also when your body repairs and replenishes itself, so missing sleep impairs your immunity and creates inflammation. When you're sleep deprived, your memory suffers—and so do your concentration, decision-making skills, and even your creativity. When we get ample sleep, the brain is able to forge new paths between neurons, overcoming injury or illness and adapting to new emotions and experiences. When deprived of sleep, the brain is less "plastic," and not as resilient. And there's a reason we call it "beauty sleep." A 2013 study out of Sweden found that other people can simply look at us and tell when we're sleep-deprived. Researchers shared that when we're not rested, others are more likely to notice our red eyes, droopy features, fine lines or wrinkles, dark circles, and pale skin. Sure, beauty is only skin deep and in the eye of the beholder, but no one wants to look as tired as they feel!

Sleep and weight gain

Sleep can definitely interfere with your efforts to maintain or lose weight, despite your best efforts. First and foremost, you're bound to lose motivation to eat right and exercise when you're exhausted. Sleep also impacts two hormones linked to hunger and fullness, leptin and ghrelin. When you're tired, your brain makes extra ghrelin, which piques your appetite. At the same time, levels of leptin drop, so you feel extra hungry for "no" reason. (When you're overtired and under-rested, your body ramps up production of cortisol, which is also an appetite stimulant.)

Plus, your body releases less insulin after you eat when you're sleep-deprived, and a lack of rest can impair your glucose tolerance, boosting not only your weight but your chances of developing type 2 diabetes as well. In addition, a lack of sleep may cause a chemical shift that leads you to crave "palatable" foods high in sugar, salt, and fat.

A lengthy study found that women who sleep five hours or less a night were 32 percent more likely to experience "major" weight gain (of 33 pounds or more) over the sixteen years of the study—and they were 15 percent more likely to become obese, compared with women who slept seven hours or more. A review of thirty-six studies on sleep and weight gain also found an independent link between gaining weight and skimping on sleep.

Even one night of bad sleep can impact your hunger levels and cravings. A 2019 study involving women who regularly slept seven to nine hours a night found that getting about five to six hours instead made them feel hungrier the next day, with stronger food cravings. (The women ate more chocolate!)

If you're quite active or an athlete, know that sleep disturbances are a red flag for overtraining, which to your body just looks like stress.

Why women really are more tired than men

Women are collectively more tired than men are—and not just because men's snoring is more likely to keep us awake. (Yep, that's quantifiable, too.) According to a 2017 study published in the *Journal of Clinical Sleep Medicine*, women experience sleep disorders at higher rates, feel the effects of those disorders more often, and struggle with sleep-related memory and concentration issues more often, too. That research looked at Australia, but the CDC reported in 2013 that women in the U.S. were nearly twice as likely than men to often feel "very tired" or "exhausted."

Unfortunately, sleep is another area of health where racial inequity exists, with nearly 46 percent of Black people falling short on sleep, compared with about 33 percent of white people. For those who identify as Latinx it was 34.5 percent, 37.5 percent for Asian Americans, 40.4 percent for Native Americans and indigenous folks, and 46.3 percent for individuals who identify as Native Hawaiian and Pacific Islander. To learn more about rest as a social justice and racial issue, I highly recommend the work of Tricia Hersey and the Nap Ministry (see resources on page 234).

How to get more sleep— and better sleep

Sleep issues are a flashing sign that you're well on your way to burnout, but it is possible to get the rest and restoration you deserve.

The goal isn't just "get more sleep," though that's a fine place to start. A good night's sleep means you awake feeling rested, focused, and ready to tackle the day. Simply being in bed for eight hours isn't enough.

Good sleepers stick to a schedule, and they make sleep hygiene a priority. *Sleep hygiene* sounds like how long it's been since you changed your sheets, but this term actually refers to habits like the following:

- Go to bed and get up at roughly the same time every day. Put the "rhythm" back into your circadian rhythm.

- Try not to sleep in on weekends. It'll only make Monday morning harder.

- Take naps if you need to, but limit them to no more than twenty minutes. Sleeping longer than that might backfire and leave you feeling groggy.

- Don't give in to the fatigue that hits around the kids' bedtime. Try to stay active between when you put them down and your own bedtime. Dozing with them or on the couch will make it harder to sleep through the night.

- Turn your bedroom into a sleep sanctuary. Close the shades, dim the lights, dig out your favorite unscented candle, and turn down the temperature. Tidying up loose ends in your space (like putting away clothes or clearing clutter from your bureau and bedside table) provides outer order and inner calm.

- Can't sleep? Have an arsenal of tools and tricks handy to keep you from spiraling over how tired you'll feel tomorrow. Here are some I like:

- *Journal if you struggle with anxious thoughts, write them down as a way to release them*

- *Lavender essential oil or pillow spray*

- *A warm bath or shower*

- *Deep-breathing exercises*

- *An eye mask to block light*

- *A sleep stories app to help you relax*

- *Earplugs to block noise (but skip these if you need to be able to hear the kids)*

Unplug Thirty Minutes before Bedtime

If I had to choose one single tip to turn around sleep hygiene, it's this one. Unfortunately, this is also one of the hardest habits to form. Thankfully, tech can help here. The Health app on iPhones includes sleep data, and you can customize your preferences to set a bedtime (and automatic alarm), get a reminder when it's time to start winding down, and automatically turn on "Do Not Disturb" until the next morning.

Electronics short-circuit your ability to get a good night's sleep. The blue light emitted by screens confuses your body's natural rhythms. Looking at your social media feeds and reading the news also keeps your mind engaged. A 2019 survey from Common Sense Media found that 62 percent of respondents keep their phones near them at night while sleeping. It stands to reason that a lot of people are walking around sleep-deprived. Tonight, take a tech vacation. An hour (or more) before bed, silence your phone, close your laptop, and shut off the constant chatter of the online world.

Why you aren't sleeping—and what to do about it

Here's a look at some of the habits that might be interfering with your R&R.

Bad habit 1
You drink a nightcap to help you sleep.

- What to do instead: If you drink, stick to happy hour.

- A nightcap sounds like a great idea, since alcohol can have a sedative effect. However, alcohol can impair your sleep quality, as it reduces REM sleep early in the night. The more you drink before hitting the sack, the more noticeable your sleep disruptions will be. So, even if that glass of red wine makes you feel like you get to sleep faster, you might wake up feeling less than refreshed. If you choose to drink, do so earlier in the evening, so it won't interfere with your rest. (And always drink plenty of water.)

Bad habit 2
You don't have time to work out.

- What to do instead: Squeeze in even a short exercise session.

- Even a ten-minute sweat session can help improve your sleep quality. Avoid intense workouts close to bedtime. Instead, try evening yoga, a walk around the neighborhood after dinner, or even an impromptu dance party with the whole family.

Bad habit 3
You fall asleep with Netflix on.

- What to do instead: Read a book—and not on your tablet.

- As with the scrolling-before-bed habit, binge-watching in bed can come back to haunt you. TV screens and tablets emit sleep-disturbing blue light, and your mind can't wind down if it's concentrating on a show. Instead, reach for a book and read a few pages before turning out the lights.

Bad habit 4
You don't go to bed (or get up) at a specific time.

- What to do instead: Give yourself a bedtime.

- We give our kids a bedtime to ensure they get enough sleep, right? So why don't we do the same for ourselves? Kids usually get the luxury of waking up naturally—but parents often don't. That makes setting a bedtime even more important. If you require seven hours to feel your best and need to rise at six a.m., then set an alarm for ten p.m. each night, so you have time to wind down. Then, at eleven, it's lights off. If that feels like too much change, start by going to bed fifteen minutes earlier each week.

Bad habit 5
You can't break your afternoon latte habit.

- What to do instead: Cut off your caffeine intake by lunchtime.

- On average, caffeine has a half-life of about five hours—but it can also stick around for more than nine hours. A three p.m. latte could be what makes you toss and turn. Instead, turn to caffeine-free options to boost your energy, like a five-minute meditation or short brisk walk. Relying on caffeine for energy means you're living on borrowed time, my friend.

Bad habit 6
You spend all day in a cubicle.

- What to do instead: Soak up the sun whenever you can.

- Fluorescent lighting isn't just awful for our appearance. Those harsh artificial lights can also interfere with our circadian rhythms. If you work in a setting where you can't tell night from day (or you work evenings), get outside for a few minutes of fresh air and sunshine as often as you can. Not only will these boost your natural energy, but the sunlight will remind your body what time it is. Then at night, keep the lights low after sunset to further reinforce the natural sleep-wake cycle. This tip is also helpful for new moms (or any parent dealing with sleep regression) to help you (and maybe even your baby) get on a more regular sleep schedule.

Nutrition and sleep

Your sleep habits can impact your cravings and hunger levels, but what you eat can also make or break a good night's sleep.

A diet that supports healthy sleep looks a lot like one that supports any other aspect of health, like mood, focus, or your immune system. Whole, unprocessed foods that provide your body with the calories and essential nutrients you need to function optimally will help you rest, just as they provide you with the energy to make it through each busy day.

If you're struggling to sleep, you'll want to consider how much sugar, alcohol, caffeine, and heavy or fried foods you consume. One 2014 study of Japanese women ages thirty-four to sixty-five found a connection between poor sleep quality and diets high in sweets and starchy foods but low in vegetables. Sugar and simple starches cause your blood sugar to spike, which also impacts your hunger and satiety hormones. Alcohol, as you've read, can make you sleepy but then prevent you from getting deeply restorative sleep. There is also some truth to the idea that spicy foods can disrupt sleep, if they cause indigestion for you, so save the wasabi poke bowl for lunch.

And then there's caffeine, the patron saint and frenemy of sleep-deprived women everywhere. The research isn't good for all of us coffee lovers. Even small amounts of daily caffeine can make it harder to fall asleep, interfere with our sleep-wake cycle, cause "rebound" sleepiness, and create dependence upon it, according to a 2007 review. The problem only gets worse as we age. A 2009 study compared the effects of caffeine on sleepiness and sleep cycles in two groups: people ages twenty to thirty and ages forty-five to sixty. Guess which group experienced the greatest disruption in sleep and circadian rhythm in this double-blind crossover study? Researchers blame the natural shifts in our brain that happen as we age.

So what should you eat for a good night's sleep? In addition to my more thorough explanations of nutrients to help you sleep more soundly (see page 223), here is your at-a-glance cheat sheet of twenty-five top sleep-inducing foods and why they help:

25 foods to include on your grocery list for better sleep

 Almonds
melatonin for regulating sleep, magnesium for better sleep quality, tryptophan for making serotonin and melatonin

 Bananas
vitamin B$_6$, magnesium, and potassium for better sleep quality

 Beans
magnesium and potassium for better sleep quality, GABA for relaxation and sound sleep, carbs for better, deeper sleep

 Canned tuna
vitamin D and omega-3s for regulating serotonin, vitamin B$_{12}$ for sleep quality, tryptophan for making serotonin and melatonin

 Chamomile tea
flavonoids to promote sleep and bind to GABA receptors

 Chia seeds
tryptophan for making serotonin and melatonin, calcium and magnesium for better sleep quality

 Cottage cheese
vitamin B$_{12}$ and calcium for sleep quality, tryptophan for making serotonin and melatonin

 Fortified cereal
carbs for better, deeper sleep, B vitamins and magnesium for sleep quality

 Greek yogurt
calcium for better sleep quality, tryptophan for making serotonin and melatonin

 Jasmine or white rice
carbs for better, deeper sleep

 Kiwi
vitamin C for serotonin production, potassium for sleep quality

 Lavender
linalool for anxiety relief and to increase relaxation and calm

 Milk
tryptophan for making serotonin and melatonin, vitamin D for regulating serotonin, vitamin B$_{12}$ and calcium for sleep quality

Oats and oatmeal
carbs for better, deeper sleep, melatonin and magnesium for better sleep quality

 Passionflower tea
Passiflora incarnata to increase GABA levels in the brain for relaxation and sound sleep

 Peanut butter
tryptophan for making serotonin and melatonin, vitamin B_6 and magnesium for sleep quality

 Peppermint tea
essential oils for muscle relaxation and sleep quality

 Pumpkin seeds
tryptophan for making serotonin and melatonin, magnesium for better sleep quality

 Romaine lettuce
lactucin to induce sleep

 Sunflower seeds
tryptophan for making serotonin and melatonin, magnesium for better sleep quality

 Sweet potato
vitamin B_6 and potassium for sleep quality, vitamin C for serotonin production

 Tart cherries and juice
melatonin and potassium for sleep quality

 Turkey
vitamins B_6 and B_{12} for sleep quality, tryptophan for making serotonin and melatonin

 Walnuts
tryptophan for making serotonin and melatonin, magnesium and melatonin for better sleep quality

 Wheat germ
tryptophan for making serotonin and melatonin, vitamin B_6 and magnesium for better sleep quality

While this cheat sheet can help you quickly choose foods to help you relax, see pages 223–31 for a more comprehensive guide of foods and nutrients to help you get a good night's sleep.

Bedtime snacks to help you sleep more soundly

Rather than a full meal plan this week, I'm providing you with a list of evening sleepy-time snacks and soothing beverages to help you rest and reset. These bedtime recipes contain science-backed ingredients and nutrients that will help your body and mind prepare for a good night's sleep.

As for what to eat during the day, you can refer to any of the meal plans and simply substitute one of these suggestions for your after-dinner snack. As I've mentioned before, the meal plans are not meant to be followed exactly, but rather to give you inspiration for what your week might look like so that you can pick and choose meals based on your time, energy, and food preferences. If you're not sure where to start, the one-week meal plan in chapter 2 (on pages 42–43) is the most basic beat-burnout meal plan.

- Sleepy Almond Chamomile Cookies (page 218)
- Five-Ingredient Chocolate Chip–Banana Oat Bites (page 207)
- Calming Vanilla Lavender Latte (page 160)
- Tart Cherry Peppermint Bedtime Tea (page 158) and almonds
- Cinnamon Pumpkin Seed Milk (page 165) with high-fiber cereal and banana
- Chamomile tea and almonds

- Cottage cheese with pear slices and sunflower seeds
- Passionflower tea and tart cherries
- Tuna and cucumber slices with olive oil crackers
- Apple and cheese
- Whole-grain toast with peanut butter and chia seeds
- Hard-boiled egg and whole wheat crackers
- Banana yogurt smoothie with wheat germ

- Steamed edamame with sea salt
- Oatmeal with blueberries and walnuts
- Cheese and sesame flatbread crackers
- Tart cherry juice and pistachios
- Greek yogurt with kiwi
- Whole wheat pita with hummus
- Warmed milk with cinnamon and honey

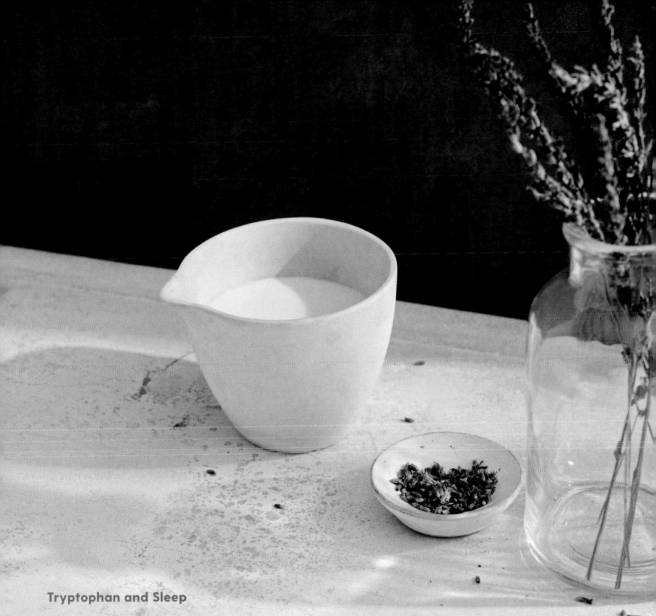

Tryptophan and Sleep

Often associated with the post-Thanksgiving meal slump, tryptophan is an amino acid that helps the body produce serotonin. It also serves as a precursor for melatonin. This pair of hormones helps you wake up (serotonin) and go to sleep (melatonin).

In addition to turkey, top foods for tryptophan include eggs, chicken, milk, yogurt, cheese, fish, nuts and seeds, and wheat germ. When you're low on tryptophan, it could impact your mood, and consuming more of this nutrient can lead to better sleep by boosting the hormones that regulate your sleep-wake cycle.

While carbs don't actually provide this amino acid, high-carb meals have a roundabout way of increasing tryptophan. A high-carb meal or snack causes insulin to be released, which reduces the levels of amino acids that usually compete with tryptophan in your blood plasma. That's why jasmine rice and other carb-rich foods are often touted to help you sleep.

chapter 7

"Good food is
wise medicine."
—Anonymous

recipes

eat

happy

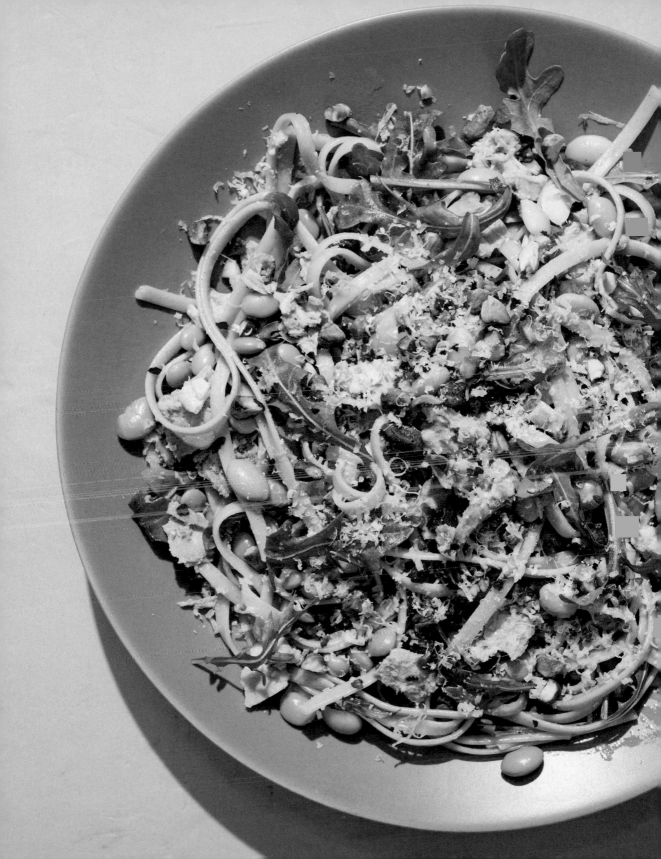

breakfast

fluffy oat pancakes
with pears

Pancakes can be overly processed and loaded with refined sugar. Not here! These hearty pancakes are based on whole-grain oats, so they're gluten-free, filling, and offer health-promoting soluble fiber. They're also surprisingly fluffy and sweet from the pure maple syrup and fresh pears. And while pancakes are a delicious brunch, this recipe is effortless enough to whip up on a weekday, especially if you measure most ingredients in advance. The batter is simply whirled together in a blender all at once.

1¾ cups low-fat buttermilk

2 large eggs

1 tablespoon maple syrup

1 teaspoon pure vanilla extract

2¼ cups old-fashioned rolled oats

1½ teaspoons baking powder

1 teaspoon baking soda

¼ teaspoon sea salt

2 tablespoons sunflower oil

1 large pear (with peel), cored and finely diced

¼ cup maple syrup

supercharger

¼ cup shelled, lightly salted roasted pistachios, chopped (optional)

In order, place the buttermilk, eggs, maple syrup, vanilla, oats, baking powder, baking soda, and salt in a blender and puree on high speed until smooth, about 2 minutes. Let mixture stand for 5 minutes. (Makes 3 cups batter.)

Meanwhile, heat the oil on a stick-resistant griddle or in a large (12-inch or larger) skillet over medium heat. In batches, pour or ladle the batter onto the griddle, using ⅓ rounded cup of batter for each pancake. Cook until the pancakes are set along the sides and golden brown on the bottom, about 2½ to 3 minutes. Carefully flip with a thin spatula and cook on the other side, about 2 minutes longer. Repeat with the remaining batter.

Transfer the pancakes to plates, sprinkle with the pears, maple syrup, and, pistachios (if using), and serve.

PER SERVING: Calories 330; Total Fat 12 g (Sat Fat 2 g); Protein 10 g; Carb 47 g; Fiber 4 g; Cholesterol 95 mg; Sodium 840 mg; Total Sugar 27 g (Added Sugar 15 g)

● Vegetarian
● Gluten-Free (use certified gluten-free oats)
● Kid-Friendly
● 30 Minutes or Less

TIME SAVERS: If you don't have pears, fold in or top with any fruit you have on hand—berries, apple, banana—or even use mini dark chocolate chips!

TIP: No buttermilk, no problem! Simply mix 2 tablespoons white vinegar or lemon juice with enough milk to measure 1¾ cups. Allow the mixture to sit for 5 minutes before using.

SERVINGS: 4

SERVING SIZE: 2 five-inch pancakes

PREP TIME: 10 minutes

COOK TIME: 15 minutes

EXCELLENT SOURCE OF: calcium, vitamin K, riboflavin, vitamin B_{12}, phosphorus, selenium, manganese

GOOD SOURCE OF: fiber, iron, thiamin, zinc, copper

supercharger

Pistachios supercharge this recipe even more by providing protein, fiber, healthy fats, vitamin B_6, phosphorus, and antioxidants.

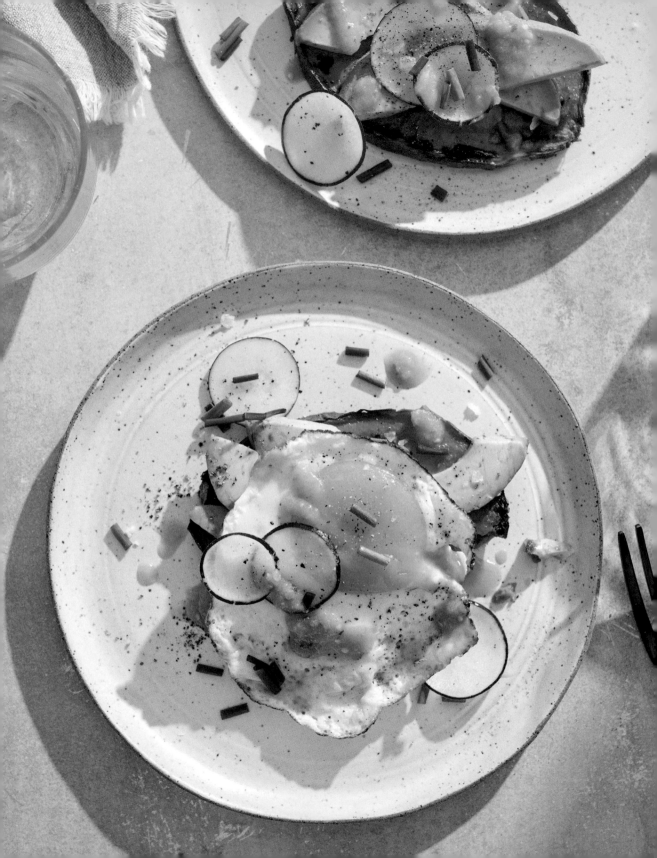

avocado sweet potato toast with a fried egg

You'll love kicking off your day with this fun flavor explosion. You'll also love getting in a serving of veggies first thing in the morning. Simply bake the sweet potato the night before. Not only is this breakfast dish pleasing to your eyes, it's good for your eyes, too, since sweet potato provides a boost of beta-carotene, an eye-friendly nutrient.

- Vegetarian
- Gluten-Free
- Nut-Free
- Dairy-Free
- No Added Sugar
- Kid-Friendly
- 15 Minutes or Less

2 lengthwise slices (about ⅓-inch thick) baked sweet potato with peel, chilled (see page 187)

2 teaspoons avocado oil or sunflower oil

2 large eggs

½ medium avocado, sliced

¼ teaspoon flaked sea salt

3 tablespoons salsa verde

2 tablespoons minced chives or chopped cilantro

Freshly ground black pepper

supercharger

2 small radishes, sliced extra-thin (optional)

TIME SAVER: If you don't have cooked sweet potato on hand, top a large slice of whole-grain sourdough bread.

TIP: See How to Bake Sweet Potatoes on page 187.

SERVINGS: 2

SERVING SIZE: 1 topped sweet potato toast

PREP TIME: 10 minutes

COOK TIME: About 5 minutes (with prebaked sweet potato)

EXCELLENT SOURCE OF: fiber, vitamin A, vitamin C, vitamin K, riboflavin, vitamin B₆, pantothenic acid, selenium, manganese

GOOD SOURCE OF: vitamin D, iron, vitamin E, thiamin, niacin, folate, phosphorus, magnesium, copper

Heat the sweet potato slices in a toaster or toaster oven, or broil in the oven, until heated through and slightly crisped (cooking time varies).

Meanwhile, heat the oil in a large stick-resistant skillet over high heat. Crack in the eggs and fry until they reach the desired doneness.

Top each sweet potato toast with the avocado and sprinkle with salt. Then top each toast with a fried egg, salsa verde, chives, and radish slices (if using), and season with several grinds of pepper.

PER SERVING: Calories 260; Total Fat 15 g (Sat Fat 2.5 g); Protein 9 g; Carb 23 g; Fiber 6 g; Cholesterol 185 mg; Sodium 530 mg; Total Sugar 7 g (Added Sugar 0 g)

supercharger
Radishes supercharge this recipe even more, as they have been shown to aid digestion, promote heart health, and keep your immune system strong.

shaved asparagus & potato frittata

● Vegetarian
● One-Dish Meal
● Gluten-Free
● No Added Sugar
● Great for Leftovers

TIME SAVER: If you can find pencil-thin asparagus spears, simply trim the ends and arrange the whole (or halved) spears instead of shaved spears on top of the frittata . . . no shaving required.

TIP: Have mushrooms on hand? Sauté them and add them on top of the frittata for bonus savory goodness and a hearty alternative to the arugula.

TIP: The Manchego cheese adds a sharp nutty flavor; however, feel free to use whatever cheese you have on hand (feta, mozzarella, Cheddar, gouda, or even gouda with truffles)—it all works!

SERVINGS: 6

SERVING SIZE: 1 wedge

PREP TIME: 18 minutes

COOK TIME: 45 minutes

EXCELLENT SOURCE OF: iron, vitamin A, vitamin C, vitamin K, riboflavin, vitamin B_{12}, pantothenic acid, selenium

GOOD SOURCE OF: vitamin D, calcium, vitamin B_6, folate, phosphorus, zinc, copper

A frittata is basically an Italian-style crustless quiche. This version is almost like having potatoes au gratin stuffed inside an asparagus frittata! You'll be so comforted by the layers upon layers of potatoes. It tastes quite rich, but luckily it easily fits into your healthful lifestyle since it features plenty of nutrient-rich veggies—asparagus, potatoes, scallions, and, if you want, arugula. Of course, you'll be getting high-quality protein from the eggs, too.

½ pound asparagus stalks, untrimmed

10 large eggs

¼ cup 2% fat milk or plain, unsweetened plant-based milk of choice

¾ teaspoon sea salt, divided

½ teaspoon freshly ground black pepper, divided

2 ounces Manchego cheese, grated or finely crumbled

2 tablespoons extra-virgin olive oil

3 scallions, thinly sliced on a diagonal, green and white parts separated

2 medium Yukon Gold potatoes (12 to 13 ounces total), unpeeled, sliced into extra-thin rounds

supercharger

2 cups packed fresh baby arugula and 1 small lemon, cut into wedges

Shave the asparagus: Lay a single stalk of asparagus on a cutting board. Holding on to the tougher end, use a vegetable peeler to shave the asparagus spear into thin ribbons, peeling away from the tougher end. Trim the tough end and compost (or discard) any remaining woody portion, and repeat with the remaining stalks.

Preheat the oven to 375°F. Whisk together the eggs, milk, ¼ teaspoon of the salt, and ¼ teaspoon of the pepper in a large bowl until well combined. Stir in the shaved asparagus and Manchego and set aside.

Heat a 10-inch cast-iron skillet over medium heat. Once it's hot, add the olive oil and swish it around so it travels up the sides of the pan. Stir in the white parts of the scallions. Then, working quickly and carefully, evenly arrange the potatoes in a couple of layers in overlapping style in the skillet. Sprinkle with the green parts of the scallions and the remaining ½ teaspoon salt and ¼ teaspoon pepper and cook for

(recipe continues)

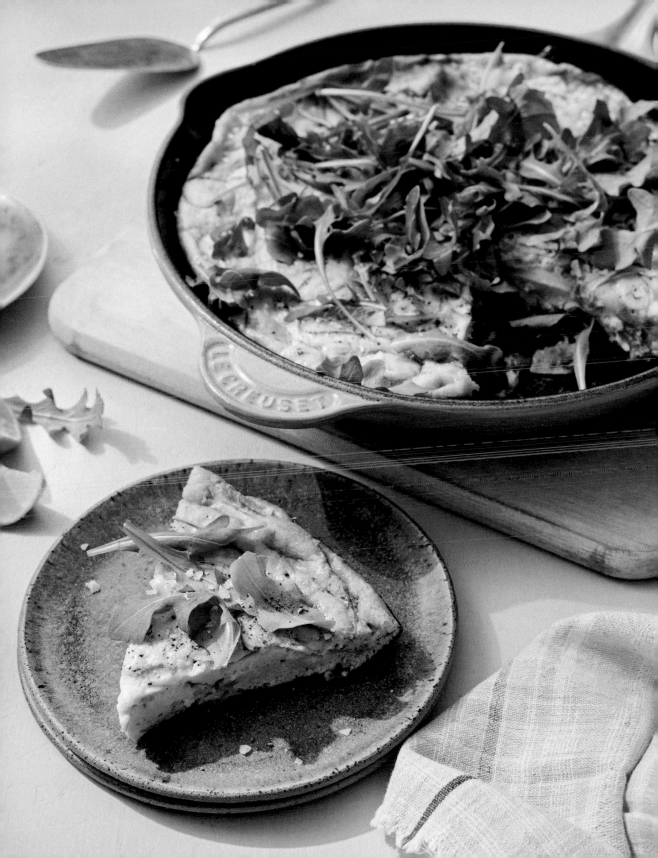

supercharger

Baby arugula
supercharges this
recipe even more by
providing vitamin A,
vitamin C, vitamin K,
folate, calcium, and
antioxidants.

2 minutes. Add the egg-asparagus mixture to the skillet, using tongs to evenly arrange the asparagus and using a spatula to press down and ensure the asparagus is coated with egg mixture. Cook on the stovetop until the edges of the frittata are just set, about 5 minutes.

Transfer the skillet to the oven to continue cooking until the top is golden brown and the center is fully set, about 35 minutes. (When the potatoes are cooked through, a paring knife or fork should easily pierce all the way through the frittata with little resistance.)

Let cool for at least 5 minutes to complete the cooking process. For best results, turn the frittata out onto a cutting board for slicing. Cut into 6 wedges. Top each wedge with fresh baby arugula and a squeeze of lemon, if desired.

The frittata keeps well in the fridge, covered, for up to 4 days. Gently reheat in the oven or microwave as needed.

PER SERVING: Calories 250; Total Fat 16 g (Sat Fat 6 g); Protein 15 g; Carb 12 g; Fiber 2 g; Cholesterol 320 mg; Sodium 480 mg; Total Sugar 3 g (Added Sugar 0 g)

apple citrus bircher bowl

If you're looking for a nourishing overnight recipe that's ideal for busy weekday mornings, this glammed-up overnight oatmeal bowl is a perfect pick. You'll enjoy the fresh citrusy aroma and the dreamy orange-vanilla combination. When you're ready to eat it, just top it with Greek yogurt, grated apple, granola or trail mix, and, if you like, goji berries. And even if you're making this bowl just for you, do make all four servings—you'll then have breakfast ready to go over the next three days.

1 cup old-fashioned rolled oats

¼ cup chia seeds

2 tablespoons ground flaxseed

1½ cups plain, unsweetened oat milk or milk of choice

½ teaspoon grated orange zest, or to taste

¾ cup freshly squeezed orange juice (from about 3 medium oranges)

¾ cup plain 0% fat Greek yogurt or Greek-style plant-based yogurt

2½ tablespoons maple syrup

1 tablespoon pure vanilla extract

1 teaspoon ground cinnamon

¼ teaspoon sea salt

for serving

½ cup plain 0% fat Greek yogurt or Greek-style plant-based yogurt

1 large apple with peel, coarsely grated or cored and cut into matchsticks

¾ cup granola or trail mix

supercharger

¼ cup goji berries (optional)

● Vegetarian
● Gluten-Free (use certified gluten-free oats)
● Great for Leftovers

TIP: For best results, zest the orange before juicing it.

SERVINGS: 4

SERVING SIZE: 1 cup + toppings

PREP TIME: 15 minutes (plus overnight standing time)

COOK TIME: 0 minutes

EXCELLENT SOURCE OF: fiber, calcium, iron, vitamin C, vitamin E, thiamin, riboflavin, vitamin B$_{12}$, phosphorus, magnesium, selenium, copper, manganese

GOOD SOURCE OF: potassium, vitamin A, niacin, folate, zinc

Combine the oats, chia seeds, and ground flaxseed in a medium bowl or 4-cup-capacity liquid measuring cup. Add the oat milk, orange zest, orange juice, yogurt, maple syrup, vanilla, cinnamon, and salt and stir well to combine. Cover and refrigerate overnight until thick and creamy. The mixture can be stored in an airtight container in the fridge for up to 3 days.

To serve, scoop 1 cup of the mixture into each bowl and top with a dollop of yogurt, grated apple, granola, and, if desired, goji berries.

PER SERVING: Calories 440; Total Fat 14 g (Sat Fat 2 g); Protein 18 g; Carb 63 g; Fiber 12 g; Cholesterol 0 mg; Sodium 220 mg; Total Sugar 29 g (Added Sugar 11 g)

supercharger

Goji berries supercharge this recipe even more by providing iron, vitamin A, riboflavin, selenium, copper, and antioxidants.

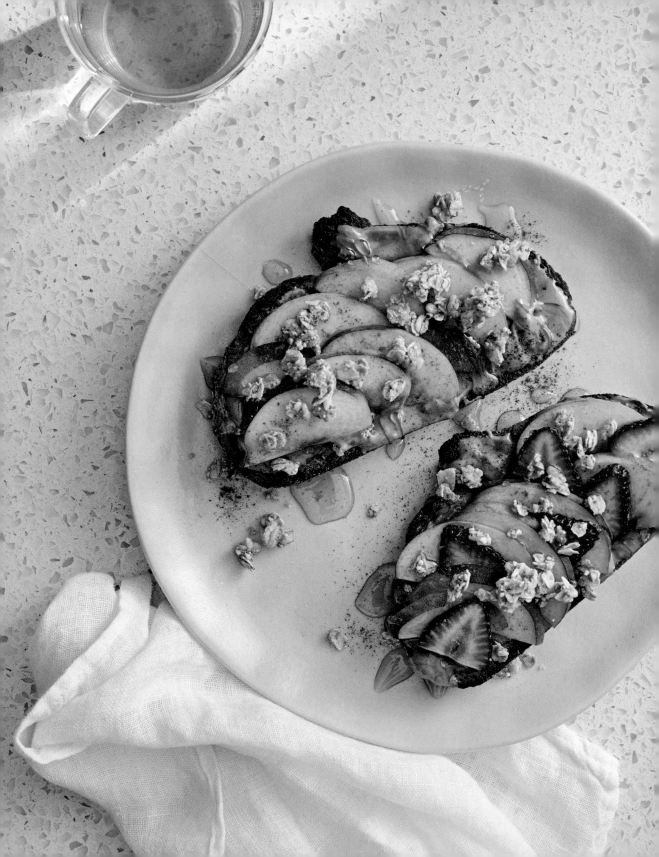

peanut butter peach toast crunch

Yes, there's time to eat (a tasty) breakfast even on the busiest weekday morning. If you have a few simple ingredients on hand, this plant-based recipe might become your morning staple. While it's a simple recipe, you'll get 15 grams of protein and 5 grams of fiber per serving for staying power. As absolutely scrumptious as it is nutritious, this peach-topped toast is a heart-friendly choice and an excellent source of fiber, vitamin E, folate, magnesium, and so much more.

2 large slices whole-grain sourdough bread

¼ cup natural peanut butter

1 medium peach, halved, pitted, and thinly sliced

2 tablespoons granola

2 teaspoons honey or coconut nectar

Cinnamon

supercharger

2 large strawberries, sliced (optional)

Toast the bread and transfer to plates. Spread each toast with 2 table-spoons of the peanut butter. Top each toast with half of the peach slices, half of the strawberry slices (if using), and 1 tablespoon of the granola. Drizzle each with 1 teaspoon of the honey, dust with cinnamon, and enjoy immediately.

PER SERVING: Calories 410; Total Fat 19 g (Sat Fat 4 g); Protein 15 g; Carb 49 g; Fiber 5 g; Cholesterol 0 mg; Sodium 330 mg, Total Sugar 16 g (Added Sugar 5 g)

- Vegetarian (or vegan if using coconut nectar)
- Dairy-Free
- Kid-Friendly
- 15 Minutes or Less

TIME SAVER: No peaches, no problem! Slice an apple, banana, or nectarine to top. For added nutrition, sprinkle some hemp hearts on top as well.

TIP: Swap the peanut butter in the recipe with ¼ cup low-fat cottage cheese or ricotta cheese for a different variation.

SERVINGS: 2

SERVING SIZE: 1 toast with toppings

PREP TIME: 8 minutes

COOK TIME: 2 minutes

EXCELLENT SOURCE OF: fiber, vitamin E, thiamin, riboflavin, niacin, folate, magnesium, selenium, copper, manganese

GOOD SOURCE OF: iron, potassium, vitamin B_6, pantothenic acid, phosphorus, zinc

supercharger

Strawberries supercharge this recipe even more by providing fiber, vitamin C, folate, and manganese.

smashed chickpea–artichoke scramble
with sun-dried tomatoes

A bowlful of flavor! That's the best way to describe this unique recipe with a memorable taste and texture all its own. Rather than eggs, you'll be "scrambling" mashed chickpeas along with artichoke hearts, red onion, and sun-dried tomatoes. A mixture of spices—which you can prepare in advance—provides rich golden color and warm, earthy flavor, thanks especially to turmeric, which offers anti-inflammatory properties. Nutritional yeast adds an almost Parmesan cheese–like deliciousness along with its B vitamins and protein.

- Vegan
- One-Dish Meal
- Gluten-Free
- Nut-Free
- Dairy-Free
- No Added Sugar
- 30 Minutes or Less

TIME SAVER: Create a scramble seasoning mix in advance using 5 teaspoons each of turmeric and garlic powder and 1 teaspoon each of smoked paprika, sea salt, and black pepper. For each recipe, use 1 tablespoon plus ¼ teaspoon of the seasoning.

SERVINGS: 4

SERVING SIZE: about ⅔ cup

PREP TIME: 15 minutes

COOK TIME: 15 minutes

EXCELLENT SOURCE OF: fiber, thiamin, riboflavin, niacin, vitamin B₆, folate, vitamin B₁₂, pantothenic acid, copper, manganese

GOOD SOURCE OF: iron, vitamin K, zinc, selenium

1 (15-ounce) can low-sodium chickpeas

1¼ teaspoons ground turmeric

1¼ teaspoons garlic powder

¼ teaspoon smoked paprika

¼ teaspoon sea salt, or to taste

¼ teaspoon freshly ground black pepper

2 tablespoons extra-virgin olive oil, divided

½ large red onion, finely chopped

4 large jarred or canned artichoke hearts in water, drained and quartered

1 ounce sun-dried tomatoes (do not rehydrate), coarsely chopped (about ¼ cup)

2 tablespoons nutritional yeast

¼ cup packed fresh basil leaves, torn

supercharger

1 avocado, sliced (optional)

Drain the chickpeas, reserving ¼ cup of the liquid from the can. Place the drained chickpeas and ¼ cup chickpea liquid in a medium bowl. Add the turmeric, garlic powder, smoked paprika, salt, and pepper. Mash with a fork, evenly distributing the spices, until the chickpeas are coated. (Note: The mixture will be lumpy.) Set aside.

Heat a large skillet over medium-high heat. Once it is hot, heat 1 tablespoon of the olive oil in the pan. Add the onions and artichoke hearts and cook, stirring occasionally, until the onions are fully softened and the artichoke hearts are lightly browned, about 6 minutes. Add the sun-dried tomatoes and cook, stirring, until the onions are lightly browned, about 2 minutes.

Drizzle the remaining 1 tablespoon of olive oil into the skillet and stir in the smashed spiced chickpeas. Add the nutritional yeast and cook, stirring occasionally, until the mixture is well combined and a rich golden-brown color, about 5 minutes. Adjust seasoning, if needed.

To serve, garnish with the basil leaves. If desired, top with the avocado and an extra pinch of sea salt.

The scramble is best enjoyed fresh, but can be enjoyed within 3 days by reheating in a skillet or microwave until warm.

PER SERVING: Calories 200; Total Fat 10 g (Sat Fat 1 g); Protein 8 g; Carb 22 g; Fiber 8 g; Cholesterol 0 mg; Sodium 630 mg; Total Sugar 4 g (Added Sugar 0 g)

supercharger
Avocado supercharges this recipe even more by providing healthy fats, fiber, vitamin C, vitamin K, vitamin B_6, folate, potassium, and antioxidants.

golden carrot spice muffins

● Vegetarian
● Great for Leftovers
● Smart Freezer Meal

TIME SAVER: Use packaged pre-shredded carrots.

TIP: For an extra fiber boost, swap in unbleached whole wheat pastry flour for the all-purpose flour.

TIP: To make gluten-free, use a gluten-free 1-to-1 all-purpose baking flour instead of the unbleached all-purpose flour.

TIP: Fold in raisins for additional sweetness, texture, and nutrition. To guarantee the raisins are soft and plump, soak them in warm water before using.

TIP: For a nuttier taste if you plan to use the supercharger, pan-toast the walnut halves in a dry skillet over medium heat until golden and fragrant, about 3 to 5 minutes, then chop and fold into the recipe.

SERVINGS: 12

SERVING SIZE: 1 large muffin

PREP TIME: 15 minutes

COOK TIME: 25 minutes

EXCELLENT SOURCE OF: vitamin A, manganese

GOOD SOURCE OF: thiamin, riboflavin, phosphorus, selenium

Ready for a muffin that has a just-right amount of sweetness and spice? This oat bran–spiked muffin recipe goes all out with spices—turmeric, cinnamon, cardamom, salt, and black pepper—making them the highlight. The black pepper in the recipe might seem unusual, but it contributes a hint of desirable "heat" while promoting the bioavailability of turmeric, which further enhances the spice's anti-inflammatory benefits. The calcium-rich yogurt in the recipe provides moistness. And the carrots make these muffins count as part of your veggie intake! Freeze several of these for a satisfying and wholesome grab 'n' go snack.

1 cup plus 2 tablespoons unbleached all-purpose flour

¾ cup oat bran

1 tablespoon baking powder

2 teaspoons ground turmeric

2 teaspoons ground cinnamon

¼ teaspoon ground cardamom

¾ teaspoon sea salt

¼ teaspoon freshly ground black pepper

½ cup mild honey

⅓ cup unrefined (virgin) coconut oil, melted

1 cup plain 0% fat Greek yogurt

2 large eggs

2½ teaspoons pure vanilla extract

2 cups coarsely grated carrots (from about 3 large carrots)

1 tablespoon turbinado sugar

supercharger
¾ cup walnut halves, chopped (optional)

Preheat the oven to 400°F. Line a standard 12-cup muffin pan with unbleached parchment paper cups or silicone muffin liners. (Standard paper liners may stick to baked muffins.)

In a medium mixing bowl, whisk together the flour, oat bran, baking powder, turmeric, cinnamon, cardamom, salt, and pepper and set aside.

In a large mixing bowl, whisk together the honey and coconut oil until well combined. Then add the yogurt, eggs, and vanilla and whisk to fully incorporate. Add the grated carrots and stir to combine. Add the dry ingredients and stir until just combined. Fold in the walnuts, if using, until evenly incorporated. (Note: The batter will be thick.)

Divide the batter among the prepared muffin cups, filling each cup completely. Dust the tops with the sugar.

Bake 22 to 25 minutes, until the muffins are springy to the touch and a toothpick inserted into the center comes out clean. Let cool for at least 10 minutes before serving.

Muffins keep well in a sealed container for up to 2 days at room temperature, up to 4 days in the fridge, or up to 3 months in the freezer.

PER SERVING: Calories 190; Total Fat 7 g (Sat Fat 5 g); Protein 5 g; Carb 29 g; Fiber 2 g; Cholesterol 30 mg; Sodium 180 mg; Total Sugar 14 g (Added Sugar 13 g)

supercharger

Walnuts
supercharge this recipe even more by providing protein, fiber, healthy fats, and antioxidants.

mains
&
sauces

sheet-pan salmon, fingerling potatoes & asparagus
with citrus miso sauce

This sheet-pan dish is not only a complete, balanced meal, it's also a celebration of veggies. The salmon fillets are petite, which showcases how veggies can be the star of the dish. If you prefer more caramelization (browning) of veggies and salmon, place the pan under the broiler for a minute or two before removing it from the oven. For extra flair and a bit of crunch, consider sprinkling with salted roasted pepitas at serving time. You'll have plenty of the scrumptious sauce for drizzling over this meal—even if you include a bonus grain side or make a salad bowl with leftovers.

- One-Dish Meal
- Gluten-Free
- Nut-Free
- Dairy-Free
- Great for Leftovers

TIP: Use tricolor fingerlings for more color intrigue.

TIP: Transform leftovers into a Nicoise salad—add lettuce, olives, red onion, and a hard-boiled egg.

SERVINGS: 4

SERVING SIZE: 4-ounce salmon fillet with veggies and about 3 tablespoons sauce

PREP TIME: 18 minutes

COOK TIME: 45 minutes

EXCELLENT SOURCE OF: fiber, iron, vitamin C, vitamin K, thiamin, riboflavin, niacin, vitamin B$_6$, folate, vitamin B$_{12}$, pantothenic acid, phosphorus, selenium, copper

GOOD SOURCE OF: vitamin A, magnesium, manganese

---

1 pound fingerling potatoes, halved lengthwise

3 tablespoons extra-virgin olive oil, divided

½ teaspoon sea salt, divided

1 bunch asparagus (12 ounces), ends trimmed

4 petite (4- to 4½-ounces each) salmon fillets with skin

¼ teaspoon freshly ground black pepper

1 recipe Spicy Citrus Miso Sauce (see below)

¼ cup packed small fresh cilantro leaves with tender stems

1 lime, sliced (optional)

spicy citrus miso sauce

⅓ cup fresh orange juice

¼ cup fresh lime juice

2 tablespoons white miso paste

1 tablespoon extra-virgin olive oil

2 teaspoons maple syrup

1 large garlic clove, minced

¼ teaspoon sea salt

1 small serrano chili, extra-thinly sliced crosswise

supercharger

1½ cups sugar snap peas (optional)

supercharger

Sugar snap peas supercharge this recipe even more by providing vitamin A, vitamin C, and vitamin K.

(recipe continues)

Arrange racks in the upper and lower thirds of the oven and preheat to 400°F. On a large rimmed sheet pan lined with parchment paper, toss the potatoes with 1½ tablespoons of the olive oil and ¼ teaspoon of the salt. Arrange the potatoes cut-side down and roast on the upper rack until golden brown, about 25 minutes.

Flip over the potatoes and push them to one side of the pan. Then place the asparagus spears, snap peas (if using), and salmon fillets (skin-side down) on the other side of the pan. Brush the vegetables and salmon with the remaining 1½ tablespoons of olive oil and season with the remaining ¼ teaspoon of salt and the pepper. Bake on the lower rack until the fish is just firm in the center and flakes with a fork, and the vegetables are bright green and tender, 18 to 20 minutes.

Meanwhile, prepare the sauce. Whisk together the orange juice, lime juice, miso, olive oil, maple syrup, garlic, and salt in a small bowl until the miso has dissolved. Stir in the chili. Set aside.

Arrange the salmon and veggies on a platter. Spoon half of the spicy citrus miso sauce over the warm salmon and veggies. Top with the cilantro and lime slices (if using). Serve with the remaining sauce on the side. Sauce will last in an airtight container in the refrigerator for up to a week.

PER SERVING: Calories 450; Total Fat 22 g (Sat Fat 3 g); Protein 29 g; Carb 33 g; Fiber 5 g; Cholesterol 65 mg; Sodium 800 mg; Total Sugar 8 g (Added Sugar 2 g)

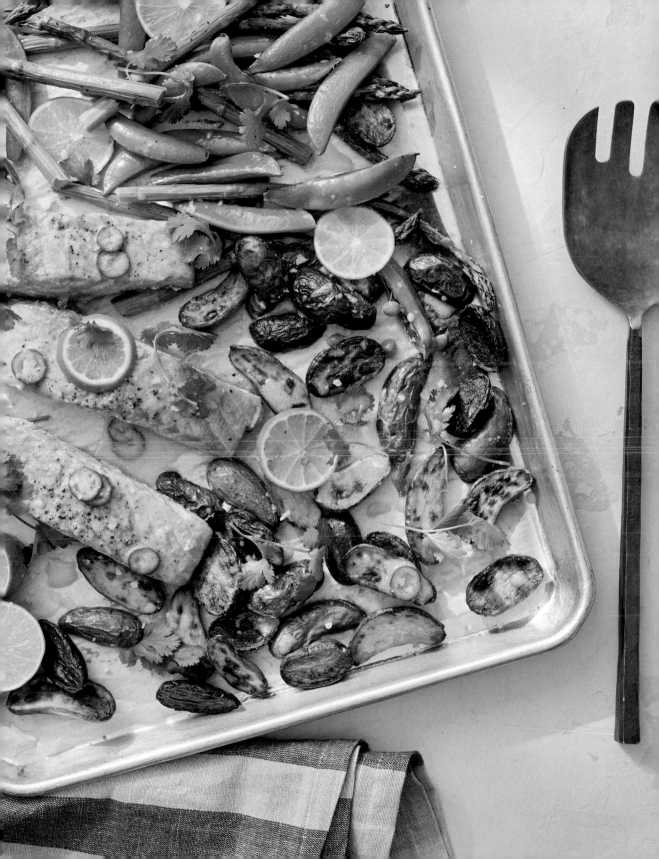

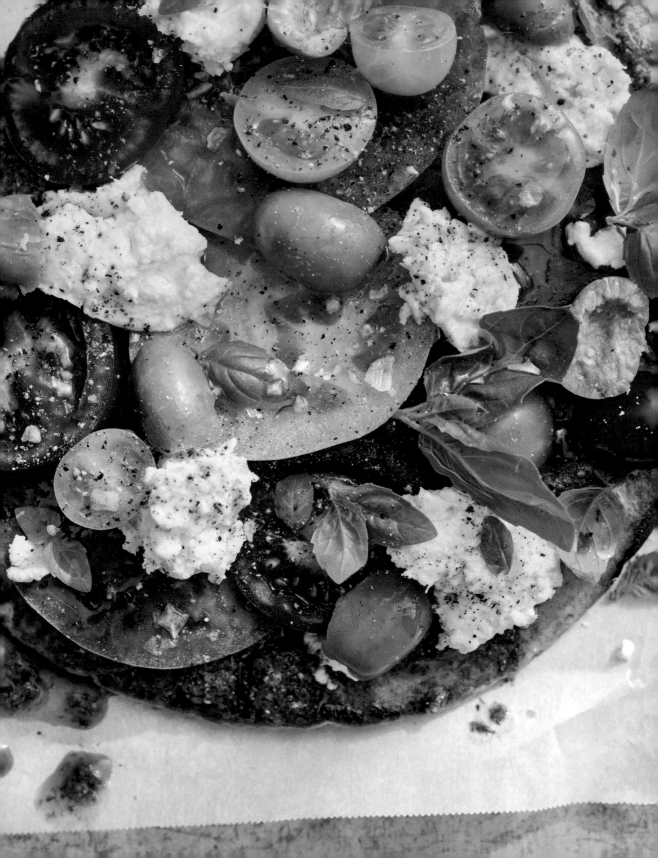

ultimate caprese salad flatbread

This is one of those fork-and-knife flatbreads to savor slowly. With fresh heirloom and cherry tomatoes, thick bites of mozzarella, and homemade Easy Basil Pesto, this adult pizza is one you'll definitely want to sit down for. And while the final product may look like a work of art, these individual flatbreads are prepped, cooked, and ready to enjoy in less than 30 minutes. Packed with protein, fiber, B vitamins, magnesium, and more, this flatbread will put a smile on your face and a spring in your step.

- Vegetarian
- One-Dish Meal
- Great for Leftovers
- 30 Minutes or Less

SERVINGS: 4

SERVING SIZE: 1 flatbread

PREP TIME: 15 minutes

COOK TIME: 8 minutes

EXCELLENT SOURCE OF:
fiber, calcium, iron, vitamin A, vitamin C, vitamin E, vitamin K, thiamin, riboflavin, niacin, vitamin B₆, vitamin B₁₂, phosphorus, magnesium, zinc, selenium, copper, manganese

GOOD SOURCE OF:
potassium, folate

PER SERVING:
Calories 680; Total Fat 40 g (Sat Fat 12 g); Protein 28 g; Carb 53 g; Fiber 7 g; Cholesterol 30 mg; Sodium 730 mg; Total Sugar 10 g (Added Sugar 0 g)

---

4 (3-ounce) premade whole wheat naan or other flatbreads

2 large (8-ounce) heirloom tomatoes

1½ cups mixed-color cherry tomatoes, halved

1½ teaspoons extra-virgin olive oil

¾ cup Easy Basil Pesto (page 124) or store-bought basil pesto

8 ounces fresh part-skim mozzarella cheese, torn into pieces

¼ teaspoon sea salt, or to taste

½ teaspoon freshly ground black pepper

¼ cup packed small fresh basil leaves

supercharger

¼ cup pitted green or black olives, halved (optional)

Preheat the oven to 425°F.

Heat the flatbreads on one full or two half sheet pans lined with parchment paper in the oven until slightly crisp, 8 to 10 minutes. (Note: They will crisp a bit more after being removed from the oven. Alternatively, rather than crisp the flatbreads, you can just warm them for 2 to 3 minutes.)

Meanwhile, thinly slice the large tomatoes; set the slices aside on a paper-towel-lined plate to drain off excess liquid. Toss the cherry tomato halves with the olive oil in a medium bowl and set aside.

After removing from the oven, carefully and thinly spread the pesto over the entire surface of the warm flatbreads while on the sheet pan(s). Arrange the large tomato slices on top in slightly overlapping style. Top with the torn mozzarella, then the cherry tomatoes with their juices. Season with the salt and pepper. Sprinkle with olives (if using), and the basil, and serve.

The pizzas are best enjoyed day of, or can be stored covered in the fridge for up to 2 days.

supercharger

Olives
supercharge this recipe even more by providing healthy fats, vitamin E, and antioxidants.

easy basil pesto

- Vegetarian
- Gluten-Free
- No Added Sugar
- Great for Leftovers
- 15 Minutes or Less

TIP: For a nutty flavor boost, toast the pine nuts in a dry skillet over medium heat, turning frequently, until golden in spots, 3 to 5 minutes.

TIP: If your basil leaves are on the bitter side, add a little honey to taste.

SERVINGS: 14

SERVING SIZE: 2 tablespoons

PREP TIME: 8 minutes

COOK TIME: 0 minutes

EXCELLENT SOURCE OF: vitamin K, manganese

GOOD SOURCE OF: vitamin A, vitamin E, copper

Pesto is considered the "yum" sauce in my household, and for good reason! Creamy, nutty, and delicious, it's perfect on just about everything. While I often use pine nuts (pan-toasted in a dry skillet for a flavor boost!), you can use whatever nuts you have on hand—almonds, walnuts, pistachios, pecans, even pepitas all work great. Full of healthful fats and antioxidants from the olive oil and basil, this pesto can be supercharged by adding hemp seeds. Use this pesto as a spread on flatbreads, a marinade for proteins, or a dressing on roasted or chilled vegetables.

½ cup pine nuts, raw or pan-toasted

2 large garlic cloves, peeled

4 cups packed fresh basil leaves (4.5 ounces)

¾ cup extra-virgin olive oil

¼ cup grated Parmesan cheese

½ teaspoon sea salt

supercharger

2 tablespoons shelled hemp seeds (optional)

In a food processor, pulse the pine nuts and garlic until well chopped. Add 2 cups of the basil and pulse until just slightly chopped. With the food processor running, stream in half of the olive oil until combined. Add the remaining 2 cups of basil and continue pulsing while streaming in the remaining olive oil until combined. Add the Parmesan cheese, salt, and hemp seeds (if using), and pulse briefly just to evenly incorporate.

Use the pesto on the Ultimate Caprese Salad Flatbread recipe (page 123) or store leftover pesto in the fridge, covered tightly, for up to 1 week. You can also freeze pesto in ice cube trays and, once frozen, transfer to a resealable freezer bag so you can thaw as much as you need at a later time.

PER SERVING: Calories 140; Total Fat 15 g (Sat Fat 2 g); Protein 1 g; Carb 1 g; Fiber 0 g; Cholesterol 0 mg; Sodium 115 mg; Total Sugar 0 g (Added Sugar 0 g)

supercharger

Hemp seeds supercharge this recipe even more by providing protein, fiber, healthy fats, iron, vitamin E, and magnesium.

poblano &
portobello tacos

These hearty, full-flavored tacos are far from an Americanized version. Avocado offers luxuriousness along with its heart-healthy fats and fiber. Portobellos provide plenty of meatiness without the meat. Poblanos lend pepperiness in a mild way. And the creamy chipotle yogurt sauce makes these nice and spicy. These tacos aren't just delicious—they're fun to prepare, too, which makes them perfect for a weeknight meal or a date night cooking session with your partner.

● Vegetarian
● Gluten-Free
● Nut-Free
● No Added Sugar
● Kid-Friendly
● Great for Leftovers
(taco filling)

TIME SAVER: Use a bottled organic or natural chipotle ranch dressing in place of the Chipotle Yogurt Sauce.

SERVINGS: 4

SERVING SIZE: 2 tacos

PREP TIME: 25 minutes

COOK TIME: 14 minutes

EXCELLENT SOURCE OF: fiber, calcium, vitamin A, riboflavin, niacin, pantothenic acid, copper

GOOD SOURCE OF: iron, potassium, vitamin K, thiamin, vitamin B₆, folate, phosphorus, selenium

chipotle yogurt sauce

½ cup 2% fat Greek yogurt

1 tablespoon minced jarred or canned chipotle chilis or ½ teaspoon chipotle powder

1 teaspoon freshly squeezed lime juice

¼ teaspoon ground cumin

¼ teaspoon sea salt

tacos

8 (5- to 5½-inch) corn tortillas

4 ounces shredded Monterey jack or pepper jack cheese (about 1 cup)

1 tablespoon avocado oil or sunflower oil

½ medium red onion, sliced

2 medium poblano or Anaheim chilis, cored, seeded, and cut into long, thin strips

2 large (6-inch) Portobello mushrooms, stemmed and cut into ¼-inch-thick slices

½ teaspoon sea salt

1 medium avocado, very thinly sliced

½ cup fresh cilantro leaves with tender stems

¾ cup fresh store-bought salsa fresca (pico de gallo), for serving

supercharger

1½ tablespoons salted roasted pepitas (optional)

Make the sauce: In a small bowl, whisk to combine the yogurt, chopped chipotle, lime juice, cumin, and salt until smooth and set aside. (Makes rounded ½ cup.)

Make the tacos: Place the tortillas on one full or two half sheet pans. Sprinkle with the cheese and set aside. Preheat the broiler.

(recipe continues)

supercharger

Pepitas supercharge this recipe even more by providing protein, fiber, healthy fats, magnesium, zinc, and antioxidants.

Heat the oil in a large, deep cast-iron or other stick-resistant skillet over medium-high heat. When the oil shimmers, add the onion and chilis and cook, stirring occasionally, until the onion is softened, about 5 minutes. Add the mushrooms and cook, stirring occasionally, until the mushrooms are lightly browned, about 5 minutes. Season with the salt. Turn off the heat.

Broil the tortillas until the cheese is bubbling and melted, about 2 minutes. Remove from the oven and top each tortilla with the poblano mushroom filling, avocado, and chipotle yogurt sauce. Sprinkle with the pepitas (if using), and cilantro and serve immediately with the salsa fresca on the side.

The taco filling keeps well covered in the fridge for up to 4 days.

PER SERVING: Calories 400; Total Fat 21 g (Sat Fat 7 g); Protein 16 g; Carb 40 g; Fiber 8 g; Cholesterol 30 mg; Sodium 740 mg; Total Sugar 7 g (Added Sugar 0 g)

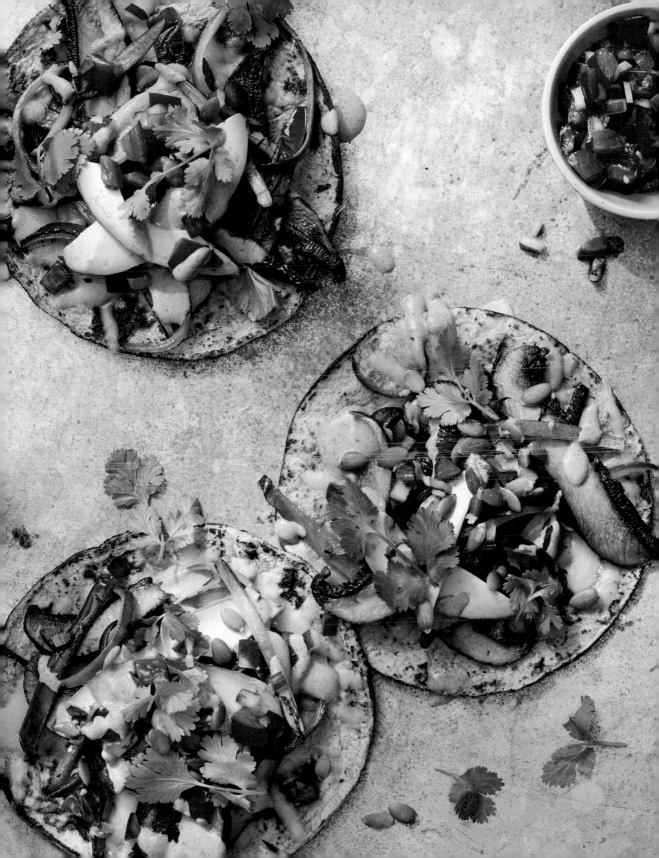

cabbage, mushroom & snow pea stir-fry

- Vegan
- One-Dish Meal
- Gluten-Free (if using tamari)
- Dairy-Free
- No Added Sugar (without Thai Cashew Sauce)
- Great for Leftovers

TIME SAVERS: The Thai Cashew Sauce adds a nice sweet-nutty flavor boost to this stir-fry, but if you're short on time or money feel free to skip the sauce; the stir-fry is still tasty on its own. Serve over 90-second or 3-minute microwavable brown rice.

TIP: For a pop of color, use extra-thin slices from a fresh red hot chili pepper in place of the crushed red pepper flakes in the stir-fry.

SERVINGS: 4

SERVING SIZE: 1½ cups stir fry + ¾ cup rice

PREP TIME: 20 minutes (not including prep for Thai Cashew Sauce or cooked brown rice)

COOK TIME: 12 minutes

EXCELLENT SOURCE OF: fiber, iron, potassium, vitamin A, vitamin C, vitamin K, thiamin, riboflavin, niacin, vitamin B$_6$, folate, pantothenic acid, phosphorus, magnesium, zinc, selenium, copper, manganese

Sautéed napa cabbage or bok choy, snow peas, and baby bella mushrooms are tossed with a creamy, sweet, and slightly peppery sauce that transforms this easy weeknight staple into a restaurant-quality dish, minus all the sodium and unhealthy fats. This plant-forward, one-dish recipe is packed with protein and fiber for staying power, along with iron, potassium, B vitamins, and so much more. If you're a newbie to tempeh, this stir-fry is a perfect place to try it.

thai cashew sauce (optional)

6 tablespoons unsalted, unsweetened cashew butter

2 tablespoons reduced-sodium soy sauce or tamari

2 tablespoons maple syrup

2 small garlic cloves, minced

½ teaspoon crushed red pepper flakes

3 to 4 tablespoons unsweetened green tea or water, or as needed to thin sauce

stir-fry

2 tablespoons avocado oil or sunflower oil, divided

3 large garlic cloves, thinly sliced

2 teaspoons fresh grated ginger

1 pound napa cabbage or bok choy, cut into bite-size pieces

1 tablespoon toasted sesame oil

1 pound baby bella mushrooms, sliced

8 ounces snow peas (about 3 cups)

½ teaspoon sea salt

2 tablespoons reduced-sodium soy sauce or tamari

¼ teaspoon crushed red pepper flakes

3 cups cooked brown rice, for serving

⅓ cup salted roasted cashews or peanuts, roughly chopped

supercharger

1 (8-ounce) package tempeh, cut into ½-inch squares (optional)

Make the sauce (if using): Place all the ingredients for the sauce in a small bowl, whisk to combine, and set aside.

Make the stir-fry: Heat 1 tablespoon of the avocado oil in a wok or extra-large, deep cast-iron skillet over high heat. When the oil shimmers, carefully add the garlic, ginger, and cabbage and stir-fry until the cabbage is lightly caramelized, about 5 minutes. Transfer the cabbage mixture to a bowl and set aside.

Return the wok to the stove over high heat and add the remaining 1 tablespoon avocado oil and the sesame oil. Quickly yet carefully add the mushrooms, snow peas, tempeh (if using), and salt, and cook, stirring, until the mushrooms are browned, about 4 minutes. Add the cabbage mixture (including liquid in bowl), soy sauce, and red pepper flakes, and stir-fry until well combined, about 1 minute. Taste to adjust for seasoning.

Transfer to bowls and serve with warm rice. Drizzle everything with the desired amount of the thai cashew sauce, if using, and sprinkle with the cashews.

PER SERVING: Calories 400; Total Fat 17 g (Sat Fat 2.5 g); Protein 12 g; Carb 54 g; Fiber 9 g; Cholesterol 0 mg; Sodium 570 mg; Total Sugar 10 g (Added Sugar 0 g)

supercharger

Tempeh supercharges this recipe even more by providing protein, iron, phosphorus, magnesium, and copper.

mediterranean eggplant hummus bowl

● Vegan
● Gluten-Free
● Nut-Free
● Dairy-Free
● No Added Sugar
● Great for Leftovers
● 30 Minutes or Less

TIP: If you'd like to spice this up, spoon on a little harissa sauce. For a protein boost, sprinkle on some chickpeas.

SERVINGS: 4

SERVING SIZE: 1 bowl (about 1½ cups)

PREP TIME: 12 minutes

COOK TIME: 12 minutes

EXCELLENT SOURCE OF: fiber, vitamin A, vitamin C, vitamin B₆, folate, copper, manganese

GOOD SOURCE OF: iron, potassium, thiamin, riboflavin, pantothenic acid, phosphorus, magnesium, zinc

For those days when you can't decide if you want to eat something warm or cool, you get both here—a warm eggplant sauté over cool hummus. Rather than serving hummus in the usual way, as a dip, here you make it the creamy base of a bowl. You'll top it generously with a freshly sautéed eggplant-tomato mixture and then finish it with fresh herbs. You'll keep the skin on the eggplant here since it adds texture, color, and a powerful antioxidant called nasunin. I love to scoop it all up with fresh whole-grain pita wedges—but you could actually eat it as is!

2 cups store-bought hummus or Fresh Herb Hummus (page 131)

2½ tablespoons extra-virgin olive oil, divided

1 (16-ounce) eggplant with skin, cut into 1-inch cubes (about 6 cups)

1½ cups grape tomatoes, halved lengthwise

2 large garlic cloves, minced

1 teaspoon ground cinnamon

½ teaspoon ground cumin

½ teaspoon sea salt, or to taste

Juice of ½ lemon (about 1½ tablespoons)

⅓ cup packed fresh mint or flat-leaf parsley leaves, chopped

supercharger

⅓ cup pan-toasted pine nuts (optional)

Spread hummus evenly into four flat-rimmed or pasta bowls (about ½ cup per bowl) and set aside.

Heat 2 tablespoons of the olive oil in a large, deep cast-iron or other stick-resistant skillet over medium-high heat. Once the oil shimmers, add the eggplant and sauté until softened, about 6 minutes. Add the tomatoes, garlic, cinnamon, cumin, salt, and remaining ½ tablespoon olive oil and cook, stirring occasionally, until the eggplant and tomatoes are fully cooked through, about 4 minutes. Remove from heat and stir in the lemon juice. Taste to adjust for seasoning. (Makes 3 cups eggplant sauté.)

Serve the eggplant sauté over the hummus. Sprinkle with the mint and pine nuts (if using).

PER SERVING: Calories 340; Total Fat 20 g (Sat Fat 2.5 g); Protein 8 g; Carb 36 g; Fiber 10 g; Cholesterol 0 mg; Sodium 600 mg; Total Sugar 5 g (Added Sugar 0 g)

supercharger
Pine nuts
supercharge this recipe even more by providing protein, healthy fats, vitamin E, vitamin K, phosphorus, magnesium, zinc, and manganese.

fresh herb hummus

The showstopper here is the herb mixture that makes this hummus deliciously spring green! My favorite herb combination is parsley and mint, but three other winners include parsley and dill (perfect paired with carrots and cucumbers), cilantro and chives (makes an awesome tortilla chip dip), and basil with a pinch of rosemary (try it with tomatoes)!

- Vegan
- Gluten-Free
- Nut-Free
- Dairy-Free
- No Added Sugar
- Kid-Friendly
- Great for Leftovers
- 15 Minutes or Less

1 (15-ounce) can no-salt-added chickpeas, drained

⅓ cup tahini

⅓ cup packed mixed fresh herbs, such as flat-leaf parsley and mint leaves

3 tablespoons cold water, or as needed

Grated zest and juice of 1 lemon (about 3 tablespoons juice)

1 large garlic clove, chopped

¾ teaspoon sea salt

¼ teaspoon ground cumin

supercharger

1½ tablespoons extra-virgin olive oil (optional)

Add the chickpeas, tahini, herbs, water, ½ teaspoon of the lemon zest, lemon juice, garlic, salt, and cumin to a blender. Cover and blend on high speed until velvety smooth and spring green, at least 4 minutes, adding more water by the teaspoon for proper blending only if necessary. Taste to adjust for seasoning and lemon zest.

Transfer to a serving bowl and drizzle with olive oil, if using. Garnish with additional fresh herbs if desired, and serve.

Hummus keeps well covered in an airtight container in the fridge for up to 5 days.

PER SERVING: Calories 110; Total Fat 6 g (Sat Fat 1 g); Protein 4 g; Carb 10 g; Fiber 3 g; Cholesterol 0 mg; Sodium 235 mg; Total Sugar 2 g (Added Sugar 0 g)

TIME SAVER: Add a couple of big spoonfuls of store-bought pesto in place of the herbs and garlic.

TIP: If you use this hummus in the Mediterranean Eggplant Hummus Bowl on page 130, be sure to double the recipe so you'll have plenty for the bowls—plus extra for snacking.

SERVINGS: 8 (yields 1⅔ cups)

SERVING SIZE: 3 rounded tablespoons

PREP TIME: 12 minutes

COOK TIME: 0 minutes

EXCELLENT SOURCE OF: vitamin K, copper, manganese

GOOD SOURCE OF: fiber, thiamin, vitamin B₆, phosphorus

supercharger

Extra-virgin olive oil supercharges this recipe even more by providing healthy fats, vitamin E, and vitamin K.

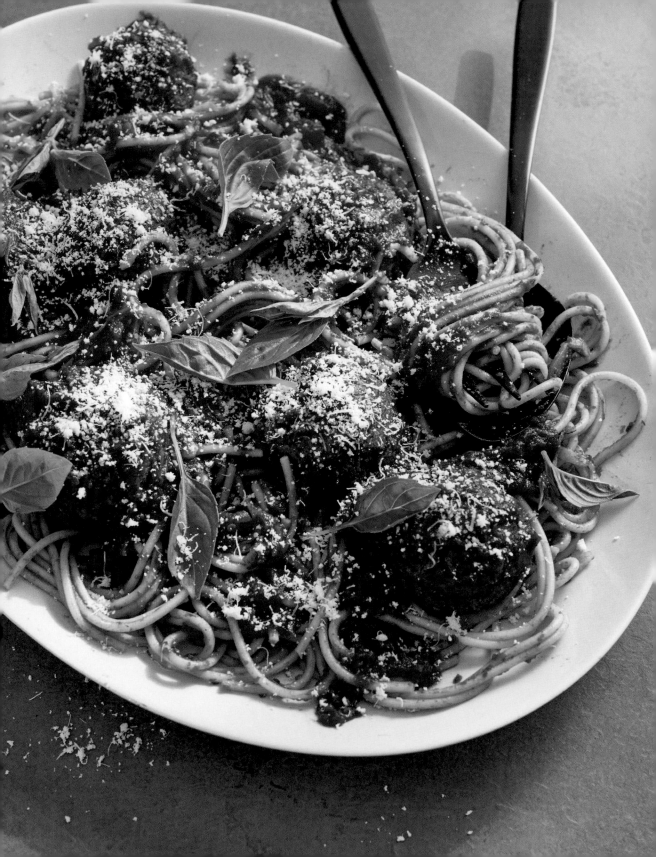

spaghetti
with chickpea basil meatballs

Spaghetti with meatballs is a comforting fix. If you don't eat meat, or if you just want to switch things up on occasion, these chickpea basil meatballs are the answer. Whether you choose to use store-bought marinara or the Three-Ingredient Red Sauce on page 135, the star of this recipe is the delicious meatballs (which you can prepare in advance, freeze, and reheat, if you want!). They don't taste like meat, but they do taste 100 percent Italian. They're rich in fiber, too, thanks to a combination of chickpeas, brown rice, and walnuts. The fresh basil and fennel seeds give them their distinctive flavor.

● Vegan (or vegetarian if using Parmesan cheese)
● Gluten-Free (if using gluten-free pasta)
● No Added Sugar
● Kid-Friendly
● Great for Leftovers
● Smart Freezer Meal (meatballs only)

TIME SAVERS: Use 90-second microwavable brown rice. Enlist your family or friends to help you roll the meatballs . . . it'll add fun!

SERVINGS. 6 (yields 24 vegan meatballs + 4½ cups spaghetti with 3 cups sauce)

SERVING SIZE: 4 meatballs + ¾ cup spaghetti with ½ cup sauce

PREP TIME: 30 minutes

COOK TIME: 40 to 45 minutes

EXCELLENT SOURCE OF: fiber, iron, potassium, vitamin A, vitamin E, vitamin K, thiamin, riboflavin, niacin, vitamin B$_6$, folate, vitamin B$_{12}$, pantothenic acid, phosphorus, magnesium, zinc, selenium, copper, manganese

GOOD SOURCE OF: calcium, vitamin C

chickpea basil meatballs

1¾ cups cooked brown rice, at room temperature

1 (15.5-ounce) can no-salt-added chickpeas, drained, or 1¾ cups cooked

3 large garlic cloves

⅓ cup nutritional yeast or ¼ cup grated Parmesan cheese

2 cups packed fresh basil leaves (2 ounces)

⅔ cup walnut halves and pieces

2 tablespoons no-salt-added tomato paste

2 tablespoons extra-virgin olive oil

1 teaspoon fennel seeds

1 teaspoon sea salt

¾ teaspoon freshly ground black pepper

pasta

12 ounces dry spaghetti

for serving

3 cups store-bought no-salt-added marinara sauce or 1 recipe Three-Ingredient Red Sauce (page 135)

1½ tablespoons nutritional yeast or ¼ cup grated Parmesan cheese

½ cup packed fresh basil leaves, torn or thinly sliced

supercharger

Reduce spaghetti to 6 ounces dry and add 9 ounces store-bought spiralized zucchini noodles (optional)

(recipe continues)

supercharger

Zucchini noodles supercharge this recipe even more by providing potassium, vitamin A, and vitamin C, while reducing overall calories and carbohydrates.

Preheat the oven to 375°F. Line a baking sheet with parchment paper and set aside.

In the bowl of a food processor, combine the rice, chickpeas, and garlic and pulse until finely chopped and well incorporated, about 10 pulses. Add the nutritional yeast, basil, walnuts, tomato paste, olive oil, fennel seeds, salt, and pepper and process just until evenly incorporated into a thick ground mixture that resembles regular meatball mixture and holds together well when shaped into a ball.

Form by hand into 24 balls, about 2 tablespoons of mixture each. Place the meatballs on the lined baking sheet and bake until firm, crisp, and well-browned, 40 to 45 minutes, flipping the meatballs halfway through roasting. (Note: Meatballs will remain soft on the inside).

Meanwhile, heat the marinara sauce in a large, deep skillet or sauté pan on the stove over medium-low heat or according to jar directions. (Note: If making the Three-Ingredient Red Sauce, see page 135 for reheating instructions.) In a large saucepan, cook the spaghetti according to package directions until al dente, 10 to 12 minutes. Alternatively, if using zucchini noodles, first cook the spaghetti for 5 minutes, then add the zucchini noodles and continue cooking until spaghetti is al dente, 5 to 7 minutes more. Drain and set aside.

Add the meatballs to the marinara sauce, gently stir to coat, and move the meatballs to the sides of the pan. Add the cooked noodles and toss with the sauce.

To serve, transfer ¾ cup pasta with sauce and 4 meatballs to each bowl, sprinkle with the nutritional yeast, and garnish with the basil.

Pasta and meatballs will keep well in an airtight container in the fridge for up to 4 days. Properly stored meatballs will keep well frozen for up to 3 months.

PER SERVING: (with store-bought marinara): Calories 590; Total Fat 17 g (Sat Fat 2 g); Protein 21 g; Carb 89 g; Fiber 11 g; Cholesterol <5 mg; Sodium 650 mg; Total Sugar 10 g (Added Sugar 0 g)

three-ingredient red sauce

You may never go back to jarred sauce once you get a taste of this simple homemade version. The butter gives it craveable richness. If you're a garlic lover, you can use 2 minced large garlic cloves in place of or in addition to the onion. If you're a spice fan, you can add a couple of pinches of crushed red pepper flakes along with the salt. If you're a basil lover, this supercharger is meant for you!

1 (28-ounce) can whole peeled San Marzano tomatoes

1 yellow onion, halved

5 tablespoons unsalted butter or extra-virgin olive oil

1 teaspoon sea salt

supercharger

1 cup packed fresh basil leaves (optional)

- Vegetarian (or vegan if using extra-virgin olive oil)
- Gluten-Free
- Nut-Free
- No Added Sugar
- Kid-Friendly
- Great for Leftovers

TIP: Use this red sauce with the Spaghetti with Chickpea Basil Meatballs on page 133.

SERVINGS: 6 (yields 3 cups—enough for up to 16 ounces of dry pasta)

SERVING SIZE: ½ cup

PREP TIME: 5 minutes

COOK TIME: 30 minutes

EXCELLENT SOURCE OF: vitamin A

GOOD SOURCE OF: vitamin C

In a medium saucepan, combine the canned tomatoes with their juices, onion, butter, and salt and bring to a boil over high heat. Reduce heat to medium-low, smash the whole tomatoes against the sides of the pan with a large spoon or spatula, and simmer uncovered until flavors are fully developed and the onion is soft and translucent, about 30 minutes. Stir in the basil, if using, and simmer for 3 minutes more. Discard the onion before serving.

The sauce will keep well in the fridge for up to 5 days or in the freezer for up to 2 months. When reheating, warm in a large sauté pan over low heat.

PER SERVING: Calories 120; Total Fat 10 g (Sat Fat 6 g); Protein 1 g; Carb 7 g; Fiber 2 g; Cholesterol 25 mg; Sodium 570 mg; Total Sugar 3 g (Added Sugar 0 g)

supercharger
Fresh basil supercharges this recipe even more by providing vitamin A, vitamin K, antioxidants, and anti-inflammatory benefits.

kimchi, corn & scallion fried rice

- Vegan (or vegetarian with eggs)
- One-Dish Meal
- Gluten-Free
- Nut-Free
- Dairy-Free
- No Added Sugar
- Great for Leftovers
- 30 Minutes or Less

SERVINGS: 4

SERVING SIZE: 1½ cups

PREP TIME: 15 minutes (not including brown rice cooking/chilling time)

COOK TIME: 12 minutes

EXCELLENT SOURCE OF: fiber, iron, vitamin K, thiamin, niacin, vitamin B₆, pantothenic acid, phosphorus, magnesium, copper, manganese

GOOD SOURCE OF: potassium, vitamin A, vitamin C, riboflavin, folate, zinc

Traditionally fried rice contains eggs; this nontraditional version does not. However, if you enjoy eggs, I designed it so you can add a fried egg on top. And if you prefer to go eggless, try adding edamame or pan-fried tofu to boost the protein content and make this dish an extra-satisfying meal. Beyond protein, this full-flavored fried rice is based on short-grain brown rice (which you'll want to make ahead of time), corn, kimchi, and scallions. The brown rice and corn offer whole-grain goodness. And the kimchi makes it gut-friendly—and quite unique. While fried rice is often a side dish, this plant-forward version can be a one-dish meal, going from start to finish in less than 30 minutes.

kimchi fried rice

2½ tablespoons avocado oil or sunflower oil

½ large yellow onion, diced

5 scallions, green and white parts, sliced into 1-inch lengths

1 cup fresh or thawed frozen corn kernels

3 large garlic cloves, minced

¼ teaspoon freshly ground black pepper

1½ cups kimchi (with juices), roughly chopped

4 cups cooked short-grain brown rice, chilled

1 tablespoon toasted sesame oil

2 tablespoons reduced-sodium tamari or soy sauce

toppings

1 scallion, green part only, thinly sliced

1 teaspoon black or white sesame seeds

supercharger

4 large eggs, fried with 1½ tablespoons avocado oil or sunflower oil (optional)

In a stick-resistant wok or large, deep sauté pan, heat the oil over medium-high heat. Once the oil is hot, add the onion and cook, stirring frequently, until it begins to lightly caramelize, about 3 minutes. Increase the heat to high, add the scallions and corn, and cook, continuing to stir, until the corn begins to lightly caramelize, about 2 minutes. Add the garlic and black pepper and cook, stirring, until fragrant, about 1 minute. Add the kimchi with its juices and cook until heated through, about 2 minutes.

Reduce heat to medium, add the rice and sesame oil, breaking up the rice in the wok if necessary, and stir to incorporate. Then stir in the tamari and cook, stirring occasionally, until the rice begins to crisp, about 3 minutes more.

Meanwhile, if using, fry the eggs: Heat a large, stick-resistant skillet over high heat and add the oil. When the oil shimmers, crack in the eggs and fry to your desired doneness.

Serve the fried rice topped with the eggs (if using), sliced scallions, and a sprinkle of sesame seeds. Serve with additional tamari on the side, if desired.

Fried rice keeps well in the fridge for up to 4 days. It can be "retried" in a skillet with an extra drizzle of toasted sesame oil or avocado oil.

PER SERVING: Calories 330; Total Fat 6 g (Sat Fat 1 g); Protein 8 g; Carb 62 g; Fiber 6 g; Cholesterol 0 mg; Sodium 510 mg; Total Sugar 5 g (Added Sugar 0 g)

supercharger

An egg supercharges this recipe even more by providing protein, choline, riboflavin, vitamin B_{12}, phosphorus, and selenium.

fettuccine
with tuna, edamame & pistachios

- Vegetarian
- One-Dish Meal
- No Added Sugar
- Kid-Friendly
- Great for Leftovers

TIME SAVER: Purchase shelled pistachios.

TIP: Choose a tuna that's low in mercury and sustainably caught.

SERVINGS: 4

SERVING SIZE: about 2 cups

PREP TIME: 18 minutes

COOK TIME: 20 minutes

EXCELLENT SOURCE OF: fiber, calcium, iron, thiamin, riboflavin, niacin, vitamin B_6, folate, vitamin B_{12}, phosphorus, zinc, selenium, copper, manganese

GOOD SOURCE OF: potassium, vitamin C, pantothenic acid, magnesium

While this is a pasta dish featuring fettuccine, all of the talk will be about the toppings . . . lots of toppings! Edamame and canned wild albacore tuna offer high-quality protein and umami—which is that savory sense of taste. However, pistachios are the unlikely star of this recipe, with their green color, crunchy texture, and, obviously, nutty flavor. The trio of edamame, tuna, and pistachios makes this a protein-packed pasta dish. In fact, it's a meal-in-one, so you don't need to think about what to serve with it.

10 ounces dry fettuccine

2 tablespoons plus 1½ teaspoons extra-virgin olive oil, divided

¾ cup shelled salted roasted pistachios, chopped, divided

2 large garlic cloves, minced

Grated zest and juice of 1 large lemon (about ¼ cup juice), divided

¼ teaspoon crushed red pepper flakes

2 (5-ounce) cans wild albacore tuna in water, drained, flaked into large chunks

1½ cups frozen shelled edamame

½ teaspoon sea salt, or to taste

½ teaspoon freshly ground black pepper

½ cup grated Parmesan cheese, divided

supercharger

2½ cups (2½ ounces) packed fresh baby arugula (optional)

Bring a large pot of salted water to a boil, drop in the pasta, and cook until al dente, about 12 minutes. Drain and reserve 1½ cups of pasta cooking liquid. Toss the drained pasta with 1½ teaspoons of the olive oil and set aside.

Heat a large, deep skillet over medium-high heat. Once hot, add the remaining 2 tablespoons olive oil and heat until shimmering in the pan. Add ½ cup of the chopped pistachios, the garlic, 1½ teaspoons of the lemon zest, and the red pepper flakes and sauté until fragrant, about 1 minute. Stir in the tuna chunks and 2 tablespoons of the lemon juice and cook, stirring, until the flavors are just combined, about 1 minute.

supercharger

Arugula supercharges this recipe even more by providing vitamin A, vitamin C, vitamin K, and folate.

(recipe continues)

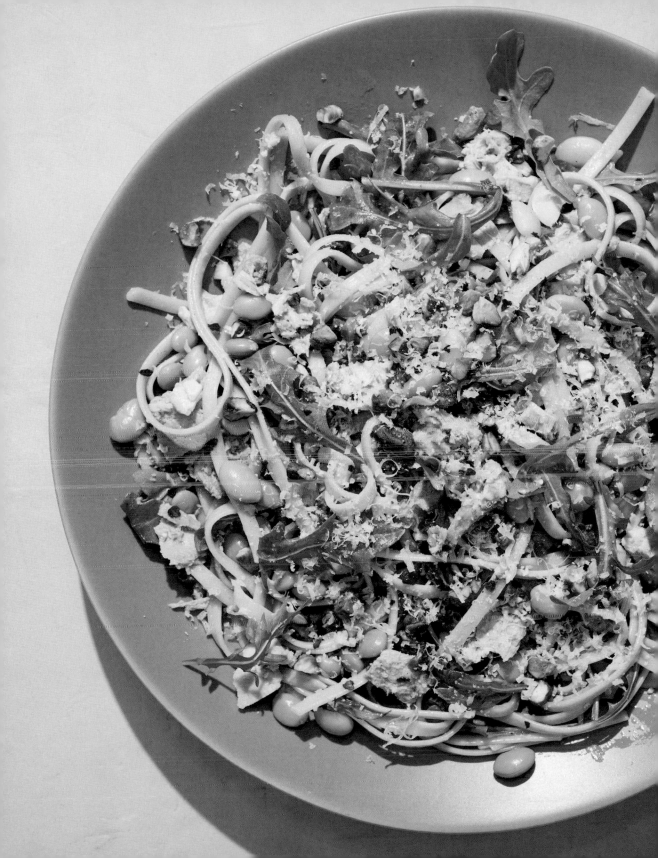

Reduce the heat to medium, add the frozen edamame, salt, black pepper, and ¼ cup of the reserved pasta cooking liquid and cook, stirring occasionally, until the edamame is heated through and bright green, about 4 minutes. Add the pasta, another ¼ cup of the reserved cooking liquid, the remaining 2 tablespoons lemon juice, ¼ cup of the Parmesan cheese, and the arugula (if using), and toss with tongs until well combined. For a saucier consistency, toss with desired amount of the remaining reserved cooking liquid. Adjust seasoning if needed.

Transfer to a large serving dish or individual bowls and top with the remaining pistachios, Parmesan, and lemon zest. Enjoy immediately.

The pasta stores well in a sealed container in the fridge for up to 4 days. Enjoy hot or cold.

PER SERVING: Calories 680; Total Fat 27 g (Sat Fat 5 g); Protein 44 g; Carb 72 g; Fiber 10 g; Cholesterol 35 mg; Sodium 800 mg; Total Sugar 5 g (Added Sugar 0 g)

smashed white bean salad & radish toast

If you're a fan of a creamy chicken or tuna salad sandwich, you'll be enticed by this open-faced, plant-based, toasty take on it. Taking less than 15 minutes to fix, the velvety smashed white bean salad is as highly satisfying as its meatier cousins—perhaps more so—thanks to its double whammy of protein and fiber. You'll be drawn in by the bean salad's freshness and the surprise pop of crunch from fennel, which gives you the opportunity to finish your toast off with the fragrant leafy fennel fronds.

- Vegetarian
- Gluten-Free (if using gluten-free bread)
- Nut-Free
- Dairy-Free
- Kid-Friendly
- Great for Leftovers
- 15 Minutes or Less

TIP: Make extra Smashed White Bean Salad to use in a whole-grain wrap, stuff in tomatoes, or serve party-style on crostini.

TIP: For a gluten-free recipe, choose a certified gluten-free bread.

SERVINGS: 4

SERVING SIZE: 1 topped toast

PREP TIME: 10 minutes

COOK TIME: 4 minutes

EXCELLENT SOURCE OF: fiber, iron, selenium

GOOD SOURCE OF: vitamin K, copper

smashed white bean salad

1 (15-ounce) can low-sodium cannellini beans, drained

1 tablespoon vegan or classic mayonnaise

Juice of 1 small lemon (about 2 tablespoons)

1 teaspoon honey

½ teaspoon celery seeds

½ teaspoon garlic powder

½ teaspoon sea salt, or to taste

½ teaspoon freshly ground black pepper

⅓ cup finely chopped fennel or celery

2 scallions, green and white parts, thinly sliced

toast + toppings

4 slices sprouted whole-grain bread

1 watermelon radish or 2 small radishes of choice, extra-thinly sliced

1 tablespoon extra-virgin olive oil

Flaked sea salt and freshly ground black pepper

supercharger

¼ cup fennel fronds, chopped (optional)

Make the salad: Place the beans, mayonnaise, and lemon juice in a medium bowl and roughly smash the beans with a fork, leaving about a third of them whole. Add the honey, celery seeds, garlic powder, salt, and pepper and stir until evenly combined. Add the fennel and scallions and stir until evenly combined. Taste to adjust for seasoning. (Makes about 1½ cups bean salad.)

Make the toast: Toast the bread. Top with the bean salad and radishes. Lightly drizzle with the olive oil, then sprinkle with the flaked sea salt, several grinds of black pepper, and, if using, the fennel fronds, and serve.

PER SERVING: Calories 210; Total Fat 6 g (Sat Fat 1 g); Protein 12 g; Carb 33 g; Fiber 8 g; Cholesterol 0 mg; Sodium 730 mg; Total Sugar 3 g (Added Sugar 1 g)

supercharger

Fennel fronds supercharge this recipe even more by providing fiber, potassium, and vitamin C.

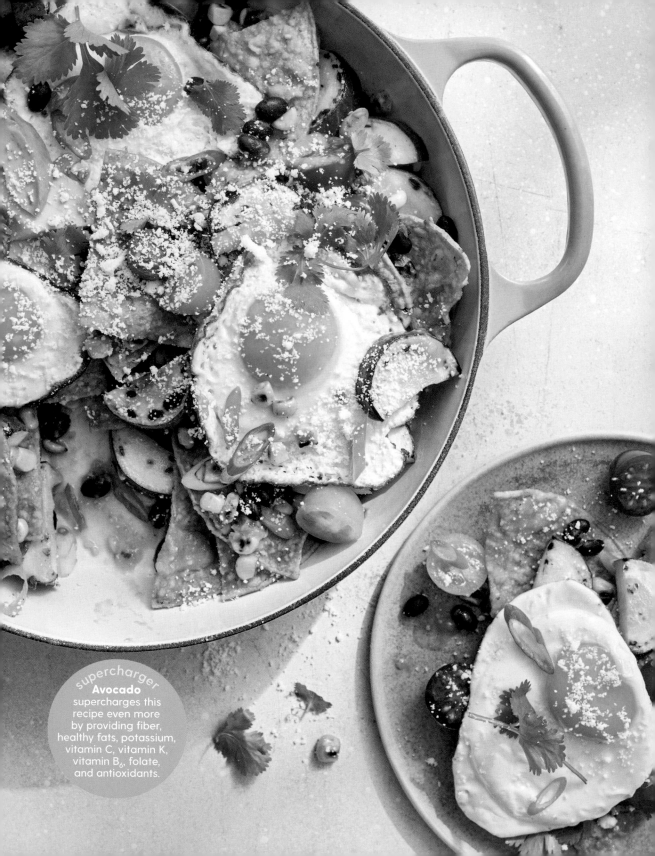

supercharger
Avocado supercharges this recipe even more by providing fiber, healthy fats, potassium, vitamin C, vitamin K, vitamin B_6, folate, and antioxidants.

zucchini & black bean chilaquiles skillet

Here's a scrumptious yet streamlined twist on chilaquiles, a traditional Mexican dish. Everything is made in one skillet for ease. Avocado is optional—but always delicious. And if that's not enough to appreciate, the chilaquiles are packed with iron, which carries oxygen throughout your body to keep you feeling at your tip-top best.

- Vegetarian
- One-Dish Meal
- Gluten-Free
- Nut-Free
- No Added Sugar
- 30 Minutes or Less

TIME SAVER: If making for breakfast or brunch, prep veggies and measure ingredients the night before for a quicker morning fix.

SERVINGS: 4

SERVING SIZE: 1¾ cups each

PREP TIME: 18 minutes

COOK TIME: 12 minutes

EXCELLENT SOURCE OF: fiber, iron, vitamin A, vitamin C, vitamin K, riboflavin, vitamin B₆, vitamin B₁₂, pantothenic acid, phosphorus, selenium

GOOD SOURCE OF: calcium, thiamin, folate, magnesium, zinc, copper, manganese

2 tablespoons avocado oil or sunflower oil, divided

4 large eggs

3 scallions, thinly sliced, green and white parts separated

1 cup fresh or thawed frozen corn kernels

1 large (10-ounce) zucchini, cut into ½-inch half-moons

¼ teaspoon sea salt, or to taste, divided

1 (15-ounce) can low-sodium black beans, drained

2 ounces organic corn tortilla chips (about 24 chips, but number varies)

⅓ cup green enchilada sauce

2 ounces shredded Mexican cheese mixture or crumbled Cotija cheese (about ½ cup)

¾ cup heirloom grape or cherry tomatoes, halved

¼ cup fresh cilantro leaves with tender stems

2 medium limes, sliced into wedges

supercharger

1 avocado, sliced (optional)

Heat 1 tablespoon of the oil in a large (12-inch or larger) cast-iron or other stick-resistant skillet over high heat. Once the oil shimmers, carefully crack in the eggs and fry as desired, about 2 minutes, using the tip of the spatula to separate eggs, if needed. Transfer to a plate and set aside.

In the same skillet, heat the remaining 1 tablespoon oil over medium-high heat. Add the white parts of the scallions, the corn, the zucchini, and ⅛ teaspoon of the salt and cook, stirring occasionally, until the vegetables are caramelized, about 6 minutes. Turn off the heat and fold in the black beans, the green parts of the scallions, the tortilla chips, and the enchilada sauce, trying not to break the tortilla chips, until the beans are heated through and chips are slightly wilted, about 2 minutes. Taste to adjust for seasoning.

Scoop onto plates with a spatula or large spoon, and nestle in the fried eggs. Top with the cheese, tomatoes, and avocado (if using). Sprinkle with the remaining ⅛ teaspoon salt and the cilantro and squirt with the lime wedges to serve. Enjoy immediately.

PER SERVING:
Calories 400; Total Fat 20 g (Sat Fat 5 g); Protein 18 g; Carb 43 g; Fiber 8 g; Cholesterol 200 mg; Sodium 770 mg; Total Sugar 5 g (Added Sugar 0 g)

simple salmon burgers
with grape salsa

● Nut-Free
● Dairy-Free
● No Added Sugar
● Kid-Friendly
● Great for Leftovers
● Smart Freezer Meal
  (salmon patties only)

TIME SAVER: Skip the grape salsa and top with your favorite fresh veggies and condiments.

TIP: Make extra salmon patties to use in a wrap with crisp veggies, or crumble and use as "meat" in tacos or burritos

TIP: Make smaller patties to serve as cute sliders for a plant-based appetizer.

SERVINGS: 5

SERVING SIZE: 1 burger

PREP TIME: 25 minutes

COOK TIME: 10 minutes

EXCELLENT SOURCE OF: fiber, vitamin D, calcium, vitamin A, vitamin K, thiamin, riboflavin, niacin, vitamin B_{12}, phosphorus, magnesium, selenium

GOOD SOURCE OF: iron, potassium, vitamin C, vitamin E, vitamin B_6, folate, pantothenic acid, zinc, copper, manganese

You can feel great about these salmon burgers for several reasons—they're an exciting change of taste from your typical patty, a great source of mood-boosting fats, *and* good for the planet! I prefer canned salmon (it's the most convenient and least expensive option), but this recipe works well with one pound of baked fresh or frozen salmon, too. While these burgers are delicious on your favorite hamburger bun, they're equally satisfying on a bed of greens or added to a veggie wrap. An excellent source of protein and a dozen essential nutrients, they put other patties to shame. My favorite part? This fun grape salsa adds just enough sweetness and heat to complement the savory patty.

grape salsa

1½ cups mixed red and green seedless grapes, coarsely chopped

2 scallions, green and white parts, thinly sliced

1 small jalapeño, minced (remove seeds for a milder salsa)

Juice of ½ lemon (about 1½ tablespoons)

3 tablespoons chopped fresh cilantro leaves

⅛ teaspoon sea salt

salmon patties

3 (5-ounce) cans skinless, boneless salmon, drained

⅔ cup whole-grain bread crumbs

2 large eggs, lightly beaten

2 tablespoons tomato paste

1 tablespoon grated lemon zest

Juice of ½ lemon (about 1½ tablespoons)

½ teaspoon garlic powder

¼ teaspoon sea salt

½ teaspoon freshly ground black pepper

½ cup chopped fresh chives (or mixture of chives and dill)

1½ tablespoons avocado oil or sunflower oil

to assemble

5 whole-grain hamburger buns

Your favorite toppings and condiments, such as arugula, Dijon mustard, and mayonnaise

supercharger

1 avocado, sliced (optional)

(recipe continues)

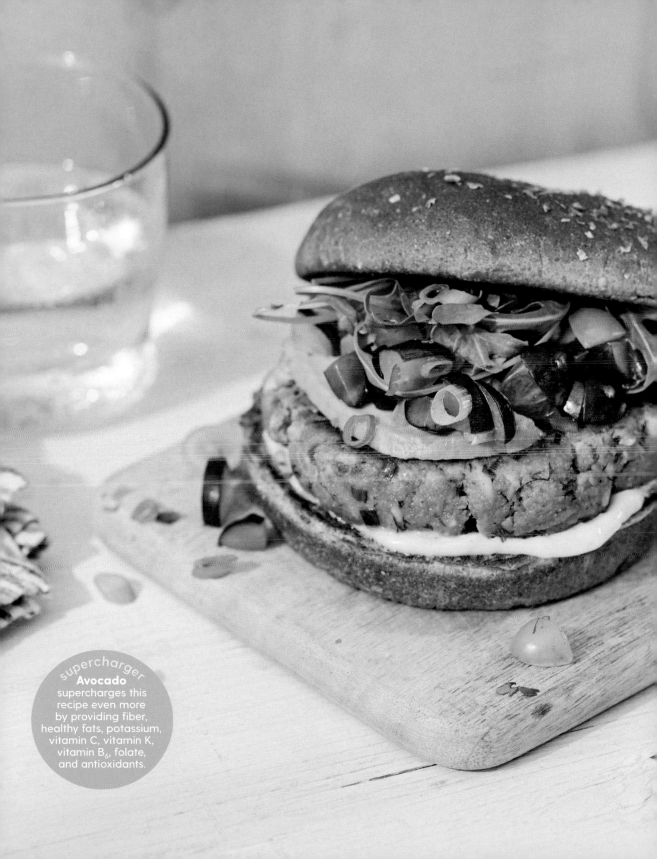

supercharger
Avocado
supercharges this
recipe even more
by providing fiber,
healthy fats, potassium,
vitamin C, vitamin K,
vitamin B_6, folate,
and antioxidants.

Make the salsa: Combine all of the salsa ingredients in a medium bowl and stir well. Let stand for at least 1 hour before serving. (If preparing more than 1 hour ahead, chill in the refrigerator until ready to serve.) Drain well of excess liquid before serving. (Makes 1¾ cups salsa.)

Make the patties: Place the salmon in a large mixing bowl and flake apart with a fork. Add the bread crumbs, eggs, tomato paste, lemon zest, lemon juice, garlic powder, salt, and black pepper and stir with the fork until well combined. Add the chives and stir with the fork until well distributed.

Firmly form the salmon mixture into 5 patties about 3½ inches in diameter. Heat an extra-large cast-iron or other stick-resistant skillet over medium heat and add the oil. Once the oil is hot, gently turn out the patties onto the skillet (in batches, if necessary) and cook until browned and firm, about 4 minutes per side.

To serve, toast the hamburger buns, if desired. Spread the bottom bun with your favorite condiments. Top with the salmon patties, add the avocado (if using), your favorite toppings, and pile high with the well-drained grape salsa, about ⅓ cup salsa per burger. Close with the top bun and serve.

Patties can be formed in advance and will keep well for up to 2 days in the fridge or up to 1 month in the freezer.

PER SERVING: Calories 370; Total Fat 12 g (Sat Fat 2.5 g); Protein 23 g; Carb 36 g; Fiber 5 g; Cholesterol 145 mg; Sodium 740 mg; Total Sugar 9 g (Added Sugar 0 g)

butternut squash
& ricotta pizza
with cranberries

This isn't just any pizza that you could order by phone. It's better! Plus, it's a fun and creative way to get your daily dose of vegetables at lunch or dinner. This recipe saves time with a store-bought pizza crust, but adds a flavorful homemade flair with roasted butternut squash, ricotta cheese, and arugula. The real magic happens at the end, when dried cranberries and lemon juice add a tart touch to make this pie truly unique. Packed with fiber, protein, and antioxidants, this pizza is as healthful as it is delicious!

● Vegetarian
● One-Dish Meal
● Nut-Free
● Kid-Friendly
● Great for Leftovers
● Smart Freezer Meal

TIP: Be sure to preheat your baking sheet or pizza stone while you're prepping ingredients so the pizza doesn't stick.

TIP: If you can find orange-flavored cranberries, they add a nice citrusy kick.

SERVINGS: 4

SERVING SIZE: 2 slices

PREP TIME: 10 minutes (not including advance roasting time for squash)

COOK TIME: 15 minutes

EXCELLENT SOURCE OF: fiber, vitamin A, vitamin C

GOOD SOURCE OF: calcium, selenium

1 pound refrigerated 100% whole wheat pizza dough or 1 store-bought pizza crust

3 tablespoons extra virgin olive oil, divided

1½ cups thin slices roasted butternut squash, at room temperature (9 ounces)

3 large garlic cloves, thinly sliced or minced

¾ cup part-skim ricotta cheese

½ teaspoon sea salt

¼ teaspoon freshly ground black pepper or crushed red pepper flakes

1 cup packed fresh baby arugula

2 tablespoons dried cranberries (regular or orange-flavored)

2 lemon wedges

supercharger

½ cup canned low-sodium cannellini beans, drained (optional)

Preheat the oven to 500°F. Place a large rimmed baking sheet or pizza stone in the oven to preheat. (Alternatively, follow package directions if using store-bought crust.)

Using your knuckles, a rolling pin, or the back of your hands, stretch the pizza dough into a thin (12-inch) round or other shape and carefully transfer to the preheated baking sheet. (If using a premade crust, follow package instructions.)

(recipe continues)

supercharger

Cannellini beans supercharge this recipe even more by providing protein, fiber, iron, and potassium.

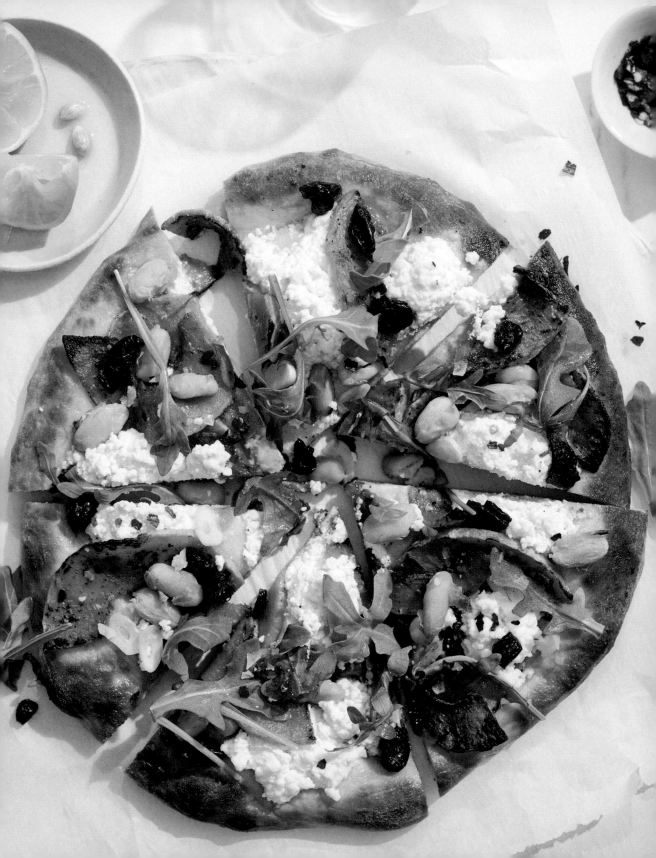

Generously brush the dough with 2 tablespoons of the olive oil. Scatter the squash, garlic, and cannellini beans (if using) on top. Top with several dollops of the ricotta. Sprinkle with the salt and pepper. Bake until the crust is golden brown and the bottom is crisp, about 15 minutes.

Transfer the pizza to a cutting board, sprinkle with the arugula and dried cranberries, squirt with the lemon, and drizzle with the remaining 1 tablespoon olive oil. Slice into 8 wedges and enjoy.

The pizza can be stored in an airtight container in the fridge for up to 3 days, or frozen for up to 1 month. To freeze, remove the arugula and tightly wrap the pizza in parchment paper, then cover with aluminum foil. Make extra for a healthy freezer meal reheated in minutes. Once reheated, top with fresh arugula and squirt of lemon.

PER SERVING: Calories 440; Total Fat 18 g (Sat Fat 4 g); Protein 14 g; Carb 63 g; Fiber 7 g; Cholesterol 15 mg; Sodium 790 mg; Total Sugar 6 g (Added Sugar 2 g)

how to roast butternut squash slices

Preheat the oven to 425°F. Peel the squash, cut in half lengthwise, and scoop out the seeds. Slice the flesh into ¼-inch-thick arches and toss with extra-virgin olive oil, salt, and pepper. Arrange the squash in a single layer on a baking sheet and roast until just tender and lightly browned, about 18 minutes, flipping once with a metal spatula.

lemony farro
& lentil bowls
with shrimp and grapes

● Nut-Free (without pistachios)
● No Added Sugar
● Kid-Friendly
● Great for Leftovers

TIME SAVERS: Swap in a tuna pouch (lemon pepper flavor) for the grilled shrimp or microwavable brown rice for the farro. Purchase shelled pistachios.

TIP: You can swap the farro for any other cooked grain, such as freekeh, bulgur, or brown rice.

SERVINGS: 4

SERVING SIZE: 1½ cups farro salad + 3 ounces of shrimp

PREP TIME: 20 minutes

COOK TIME: 35 minutes

EXCELLENT SOURCE OF: fiber, iron, potassium, thiamin, vitamin B_6, folate, vitamin B_{12}, pantothenic acid, phosphorus, zinc, selenium, copper, manganese

GOOD SOURCE OF: calcium, vitamin A, vitamin C, vitamin E, vitamin K, niacin, magnesium

This fragrant and filling salad is full of taste *and* texture. Not only do farro and lentils make this dish hearty and comforting, they offer fiber and protein to keep you satisfied and energized, too. Red grapes add a tasty pop of natural sweetness to balance out the saltiness of green olives, and the supercharger pistachios give a fun and nutritious crunch, if you choose to use them! While this recipe works perfect as a side dish, pan-seared shrimp make it a complete meal for a busy weeknight or date-night dinner.

farro salad

1¼ cups dry farro

1 tablespoon grated lemon zest

Juice of 1 large lemon (about ¼ cup)

2 teaspoons honey

1 large garlic clove, minced

¼ teaspoon sea salt, or to taste

½ teaspoon freshly ground black pepper

¼ cup extra-virgin olive oil

1 cup red seedless grapes, halved

1 cup canned lentils, drained

½ cup pitted Castelvetrano olives, finely chopped or thinly sliced

2 cups packed baby arugula (2 ounces)

pan-seared shrimp

12 ounces shrimp, with or without tails, peeled and deveined

¼ teaspoon sea salt

¼ teaspoon freshly ground black pepper

1 tablespoon extra-virgin olive oil or butter

supercharger

⅓ cup salted, roasted pistachios, chopped, divided (optional)

Make the farro: Bring a medium saucepan of water to a boil. Add the farro, reduce heat to low, and simmer uncovered until tender, about 30 minutes or per package directions. Drain and set aside. (Makes 3 cups cooked farro.)

While the farro is simmering, prepare the dressing: In a large mixing or serving bowl, whisk together the lemon zest and juice, honey, garlic, salt, and pepper. Slowly stream in the olive oil, whisking until combined. Add the warm (or room-temperature) farro and stir to combine. Then

(recipe continues)

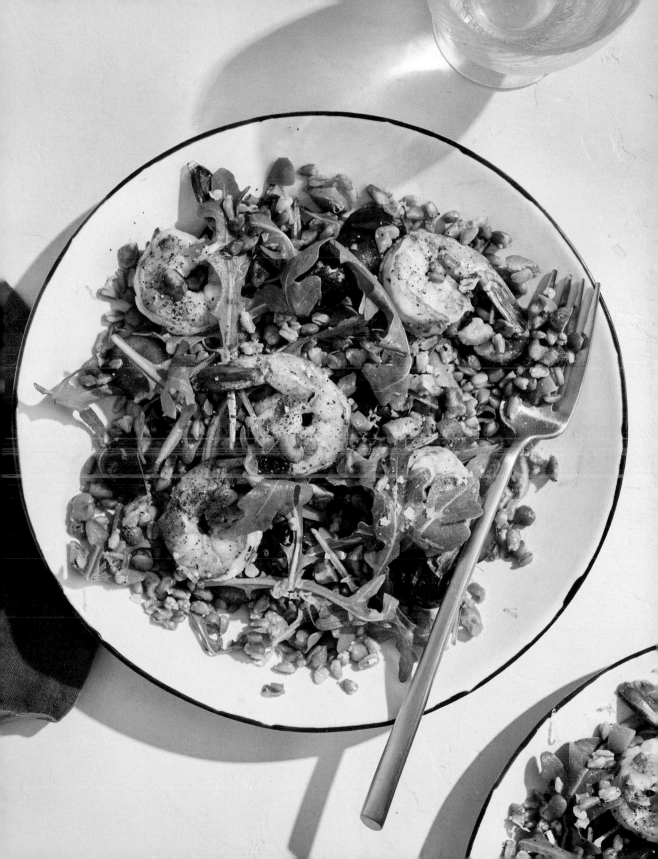

supercharger

Pistachios
supercharge this
recipe even more by
providing protein, fiber,
healthy fats, vitamin B_6,
phosphorus, and
antioxidants.

add the grapes, lentils, olives, arugula, and half of the pistachio (if using), and stir to combine. Taste to adjust for seasoning. Set aside or transfer the farro salad to individual bowls.

Make the shrimp: Pat the shrimp dry with paper towels. Season with the salt and pepper. Heat the oil in a large skillet over medium heat. Once it shimmers, add the shrimp and cook undisturbed until opaque and cooked through, about 2 to 3 minutes per side. Transfer to a plate and set aside.

Top the farro salad with the shrimp and garnish with the remaining chopped pistachios, if using. Serve as is or chilled as a salad.

Bowls keep well covered in the fridge for up to 2 days.

PER SERVING: Calories 580; Total Fat 21 g (Sat Fat 3 g); Protein 29 g; Carb 72 g; Fiber 13 g; Cholesterol 105 mg; Sodium 800 mg; Total Sugar 9 g (Added Sugar 3 g)

fig & gruyère panini

For those nights when you simply can't muster up the energy to cook but want something tasty, this panini is the perfect comfort food solution. Gruyère is an ideal full-flavored cheese to use in this panini, and couples beautifully with the sweet figs, but if you want to change things up on occasion, enjoy it with provolone, fontina, mozzarella, or Gorgonzola. Unlike a greasy grilled cheese, this sandwich is packed with nutrient-dense, soft baby greens. Add the fresh basil for an additional punch of flavor and nutrition. Planning to feed four? This recipe can be easily doubled.

- Vegetarian
- Nut-Free
- No Added Sugar
- Kid-Friendly
- 15 Minutes or Less

TIP: For the ultimate comfort food pairing, enjoy this with the Sweet Potato, Tomato, & Turmeric Soup on page 168.

TIP: If it's not fig season, substitute ¾ cup thinly sliced peaches, pears, or apples.

SERVINGS: 2

SERVING SIZE: 1 sandwich

PREP TIME: 10 minutes

COOK TIME: 5 minutes

EXCELLENT SOURCE OF: fiber, calcium, vitamin A, vitamin C, vitamin K, vitamin B$_{12}$, phosphorus, copper

GOOD SOURCE OF: iron, riboflavin, vitamin B$_6$, pantothenic acid, magnesium, zinc, selenium, manganese

2½ ounces Gruyère, extra-thinly sliced

4 thick (1.5-ounce) slices rustic whole-grain bread

3 large or 4 medium fresh black Mission figs, thinly sliced

¼ teaspoon freshly ground black pepper

¼ teaspoon sea salt, divided

1½ teaspoons balsamic vinegar

1 teaspoon extra-virgin olive oil

1¼ cups packed fresh baby kale (1.25 ounces)

1 tablespoon minced red onion

supercharger

10 large fresh basil leaves (optional)

Heat the panini press to medium-high heat.

On a cutting board, arrange the Gruyère on all four bread slices. Top two of the slices with the basil (if using), and figs. Sprinkle with the black pepper and ⅛ teaspoon of the salt. Set aside.

In a medium bowl, whisk together the balsamic vinegar, olive oil, and the remaining ⅛ teaspoon salt. Add the baby kale and onion and toss to coat.

Add the baby kale salad on top of the two fig-topped bread slices. Then firmly place the remaining cheese-topped bread slices on top, cheese-side down, to form a sandwich.

Grill both of the paninis at once, with the lid closed, until the cheese is melted and the bread is toasted, 4 to 5 minutes.

PER SERVING: Calories 470; Total Fat 19 g (Sat Fat 7 g); Protein 20 g; Carb 60 g; Fiber 12 g; Cholesterol 40 mg; Sodium 770 mg; Total Sugar 23 g (Added Sugar 0 g)

supercharger
Fresh basil supercharges this recipe even more by providing vitamin A, vitamin K, antioxidants, and anti-inflammatory benefits.

beverages

turmeric hot cocoa

This fancy hot cocoa beverage will warm you up from the inside out—and it takes only 10 minutes to make! Unsweetened cocoa powder, honey, and pure vanilla extract give this drink its traditional hot cocoa taste, while anti-inflammatory spices like cinnamon, ginger, and turmeric make it equal parts nourishing and satisfying. A twist of black pepper unleashes the medicinal properties of turmeric, while ground cinnamon has been shown to calm sugar cravings and boost mental performance. If you've got leftovers, enjoy as a chilled cocoa. Or transform it into the coolest ever ice cream flavor if you've got an ice cream maker.

● Vegetarian
● Gluten-Free
● Nut-Free
● Dairy-Free
● Kid-Friendly
● 15 Minutes or Less

SERVINGS: 4

SERVING SIZE: about 1 cup each

PREP TIME: 5 minutes

COOK TIME: 5 minutes

EXCELLENT SOURCE OF: fiber, vitamin D, calcium, vitamin A, riboflavin, vitamin B$_{12}$, phosphorus, copper, manganese

GOOD SOURCE OF: iron, potassium, magnesium

4 cups oat milk or milk of choice

⅓ cup unsweetened cocoa powder

2 teaspoons ground turmeric

1 teaspoon ground cinnamon

¼ teaspoon ground ginger

⅛ teaspoon freshly ground black pepper

3 tablespoons honey

2 teaspoons unrefined (virgin) coconut oil

1 teaspoon pure vanilla extract

supercharger

4 cinnamon sticks (optional)

Place all of the ingredients in a high-powered blender. Blend on high until smooth and creamy, about 30 seconds. Pour the cocoa mixture into a medium saucepan over medium-high heat and cook, whisking occasionally, until the mixture is simmering hot (not boiling), about 5 minutes.

Pour the hot cocoa into mugs, top with cinnamon sticks, if using, and enjoy!

PER SERVING: Calories 210; Total Fat 8 g (Sat Fat 3 g); Protein 5 g; Carb 35 g; Fiber 5 g; Cholesterol 0 mg; Sodium 105 mg; Total Sugar 20 g (Added Sugar 13 g)

supercharger

Cinnamon sticks supercharge this recipe even more by providing antioxidants and anti-inflammatory properties.

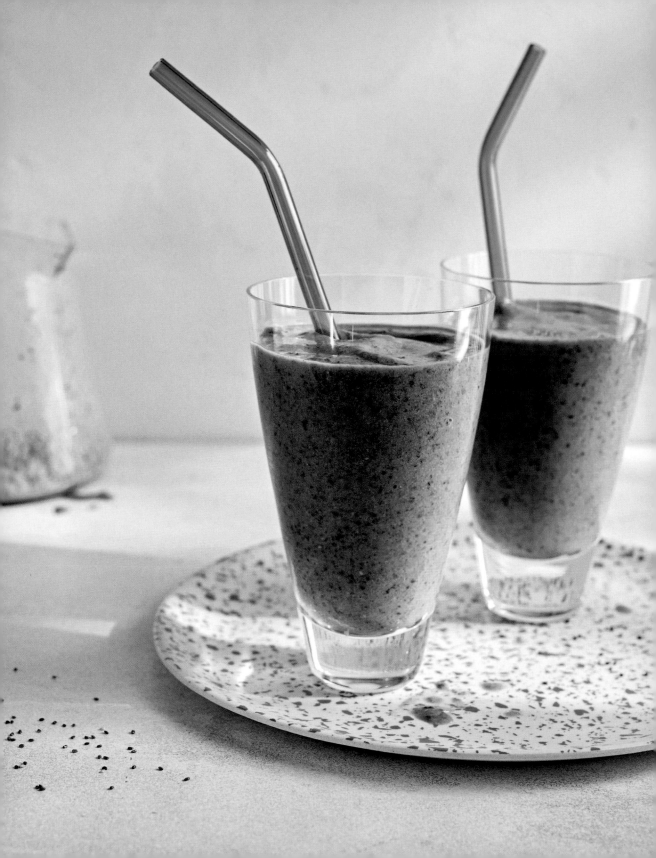

pomegranate, mandarin & ginger smoothie

This smoothie tastes like a tropical breeze with a California twist, thanks to the refreshing mandarin oranges and antioxidant-rich pomegranate juice! Frozen bananas give this smoothie its creamy texture, while the mandarin orange pulp adds an intriguing texture, along with an extra dose of fiber and vitamin C. The ginger and walnuts add to its healthfulness and unique flair, and you can supercharge it by adding chia seeds. While I love this smoothie as is, you can also add a splash of rum to transform it into a frozen daiquiri!

- Vegan
- Gluten-Free
- Dairy-Free
- No Added Sugar
- Kid-Friendly
- 15 Minutes or Less

SERVINGS: 4

SERVING SIZE: 1 cup

PREP TIME: 8 minutes (plus banana freezing time)

COOK TIME: 0 minutes

EXCELLENT SOURCE OF: vitamin A, vitamin C, vitamin B$_6$, copper, manganese

GOOD SOURCE OF: fiber, potassium, folate, pantothenic acid, magnesium

¾ cup 100% pomegranate juice

½ teaspoon grated mandarin orange zest (from about 1 mandarin orange)

4 whole mandarin oranges, peeled and halved

2 large ripe bananas, peeled, each broken into 4 pieces and frozen

¼ cup raw walnut pieces

½ cup ice or 4 ice cubes

1 teaspoon grated fresh ginger

supercharger

2 tablespoons chia seeds (optional)

Place all of the ingredients in a high-powered blender. Process on high until smooth and creamy, about 1 minute.

Pour into 4 chilled glasses and enjoy immediately!

PER SERVING: Calories 180; Total Fat 5 g (Sat Fat 0.5 g); Protein 3 g; Carb 35 g; Fiber 4 g; Cholesterol 0 mg; Sodium 5 mg; Total Sugar 24 g (Added Sugar 0 g)

supercharger

Chia seeds supercharge this recipe even more by providing protein, fiber, healthy fats, calcium, phosphorus, and magnesium.

tart cherry peppermint bedtime tea

- Vegetarian
- Gluten-Free
- Nut-Free
- Dairy-Free
- 15 Minutes or Less

TIME SAVER: It's fine to prepare this in your microwave.

TIP: Using oat milk instead of water not only adds a boost of nutrition, it creates a creamier version and turns a pretty deep mauve color.

SERVINGS: 2

SERVING SIZE: ¾ cup

PREP TIME: 5 minutes

COOK TIME: 5 minutes

Need to catch some Z's? This clever cup of tea may just help—and there's science to support it! First, you'll be using caffeine-free peppermint tea. Research suggests that bioactive compounds in peppermint may help with relaxation and improve sleep quality. But you won't just be steeping the peppermint tea in plain water; you'll use tart cherry juice, too. Tart cherries contain naturally occurring melatonin, which may be beneficial for improving both sleep quality and sleep duration. What's more, this peaceful brewed cup of evening delight is tart with just enough sweetness to please your palate. Wishing you sweet (tart!) dreams.

¾ cup Montmorency tart cherry juice

¾ cup water

2 peppermint tea bags

2 teaspoons honey

2 fresh mint sprigs

supercharger

swap in ¾ cup plain unsweetened oat milk for the water (optional)

In a small saucepan or teakettle, combine the tart cherry juice with ¾ cup water (or oat milk, if supercharging) and bring just to a boil over high heat. Add the tea bags, turn off the heat, and steep for 5 minutes or until the tea has reached the desired strength. Stir in the honey and garnish with the mint sprigs. Serve warm.

PER SERVING: Calories 70; Total Fat 0 g (Sat Fat 0 g); Protein 0 g; Carb 18 g; Fiber 0 g; Cholesterol 0 mg; Sodium 10 mg; Total Sugar 15 g (Added Sugar 6 g)

supercharger

Fortified oat milk supercharges this recipe even more by providing vitamin D, calcium, riboflavin, vitamin B_{12}, and phosphorus.

blueberry cacao smoothie

supercharger

Cacao nibs
supercharge this recipe even more by providing fiber, magnesium, and antioxidants.

The vivid purple color is a feast for your eyes; the flavor is a treat for your taste buds . . . including the crunchy bits of cacao nibs, if you choose to supercharge it. While this smoothie is designed as a dessert or a snack, you could enjoy it as a light breakfast in a pinch, as it's an excellent source of both protein and fiber for staying power. The combo of blueberries and cacao is not just a winning flavor duo, it also provides a powerhouse of health-promoting antioxidants. Plus, the sneaky cauliflower makes it extra creamy—and extra nutritious!

- Vegan (without honey)
- Gluten-Free
- Nut-Free
- Dairy-Free
- No Added Sugar (without honey)
- Kid-Friendly
- Great for Leftovers
- 15 Minutes or Less

1 cup frozen blueberries, plus more for garnish

1 large ripe banana, peeled, sliced, and frozen

½ cup frozen cauliflower

1½ cups plain unsweetened soy milk or milk of choice

¼ cup unsweetened cacao powder

2 tablespoons 100% fruit-sweetened (no-sugar-added) blueberry jam or 2 teaspoons honey

½ teaspoon pure vanilla extract

⅛ teaspoon sea salt (optional)

supercharger

2 tablespoons cacao nibs (optional)

Place the blueberries, banana, cauliflower, soy milk, cacao powder, jam, vanilla, salt (if using), and 1 tablespoon cacao nibs (if using) in a blender. Cover and process on high speed until smooth, about 2 minutes.

Pour into two large chilled glasses and garnish with a few extra blueberries and the remaining 1 tablespoon cacao nibs (if using).

PER SERVING: Calories 220, Total Fat 5 g (Sat Fat 1.5 g); Protein 10 g; Carb 44 g; Fiber 11 g; Cholesterol 0 mg; Sodium 170 mg; Total Sugar 20 g (Added Sugar 0 g)

TIME SAVER: Measure out all of the frozen ingredients in advance and store them together in a sealable freezer container or zip-top bag.

TIP: Because you're using frozen produce as the "ice" for this smoothie, it doesn't get watery as it sits. That means you can make it in advance and keep it chilled in the fridge.

SERVINGS: 2

SERVING SIZE: 1⅔ cups

PREP TIME: 8 minutes (not including produce freezing time)

COOK TIME: 0 minutes

EXCELLENT SOURCE OF: fiber, calcium, vitamin C, riboflavin, vitamin B_6, folate, vitamin B_{12}, phosphorus, magnesium, copper, manganese

GOOD SOURCE OF: vitamin D, iron, potassium, vitamin A, vitamin K, zinc, selenium

calming vanilla lavender latte

- Vegetarian (or vegan if using coconut nectar)
- Gluten-Free
- Dairy-Free
- 15 Minutes or Less

SERVINGS: 2

SERVING SIZE: 1⅓ cups, or 1¾ cups with froth after blending in the cashews

PREP TIME: 5 minutes

COOK TIME: 10 minutes

EXCELLENT SOURCE OF: vitamin D, calcium, vitamin A, riboflavin, vitamin B₁₂, phosphorus

GOOD SOURCE OF: fiber, potassium

Lattes don't need to give you the jitters. This lovely coffee-free latte is based on oat milk and dried lavender buds. Preliminary research suggests that a compound in lavender called linalool may play a role in reducing anxiety levels. Good news, right? If you're not familiar with them, lavender buds can be found in the spice aisle or bulk section of natural foods markets. The comforting combination of floral and vanilla aromas in this latte is so soothing—it even looks soothing, especially after blending in the creamy cashews.

3 cups plain unsweetened oat milk or milk of choice

1 tablespoon plus ¼ teaspoon dry lavender buds, divided

1 tablespoon plus 1 teaspoon honey or coconut nectar

1 teaspoon unrefined (virgin) coconut oil

½ teaspoon pure vanilla extract

supercharger

3 tablespoons unsalted whole cashews (optional)

In a medium saucepan, bring the oat milk and 1 tablespoon of the lavender buds to a gentle simmer over medium heat. (You should see active bubbles around the edges of the saucepan and get a lavender aroma.) Reduce the heat to low and let steep for 5 minutes. Pour through a fine-mesh strainer and compost (or discard) the lavender.

Return the lavender-infused milk to the saucepan. Stir in the honey, coconut oil, and vanilla and heat for another 2 minutes over low heat. Serve as is, or enjoy a frothed version by transferring the lavender milk to a high-powered blender and blending on high for 20 seconds. If using, blend the cashews into the milk for 1 minute on high, until creamy. Transfer to two mugs, sprinkle with the remaining ¼ teaspoon lavender buds, and enjoy immediately.

PER SERVING: Calories 250; Total Fat 10 g (Sat Fat 2.5 g); Protein 5 g; Carb 36 g; Fiber 3 g; Cholesterol 0 mg; Sodium 150 mg; Total Sugar 22 g (Added Sugar 11 g)

supercharger
Cashews supercharge this recipe even more by providing protein, healthy fats, vitamin K, phosphorus, magnesium, zinc, copper, and manganese.

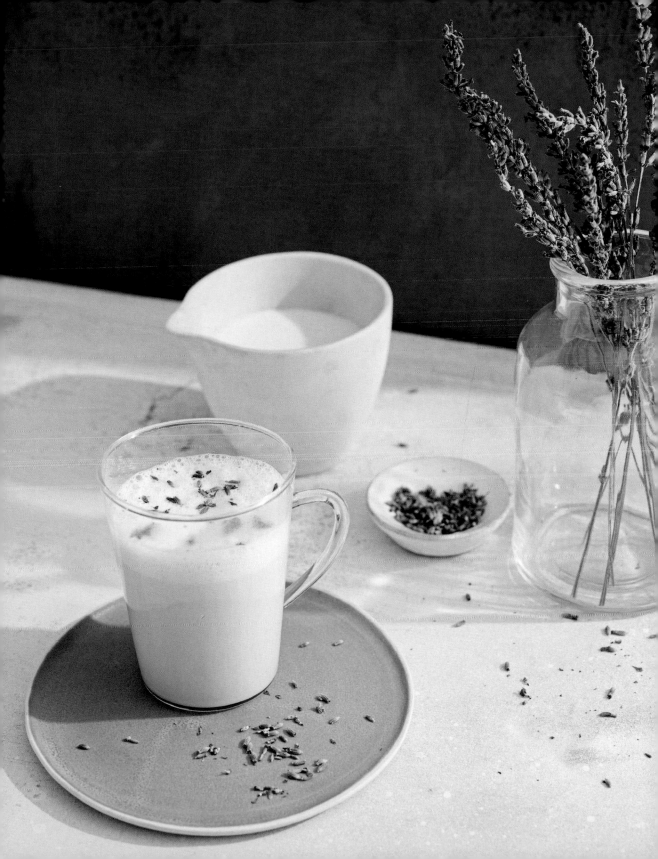

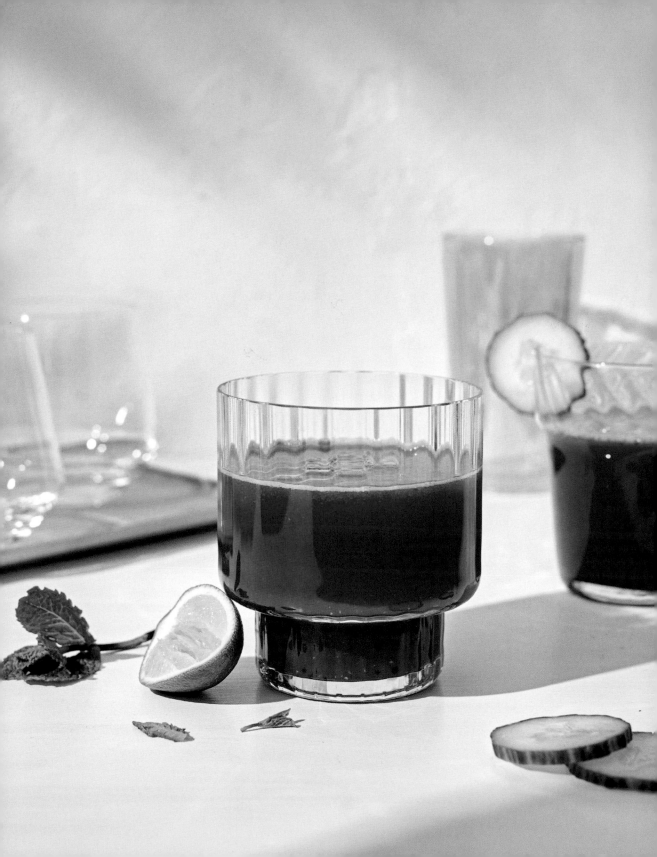

watermelon cucumber juice

This is such a refreshing summery beverage. Close your eyes as you sip it and you'll feel like you're on a luxurious spa trip. Add real ginger ale or ginger beer (alcohol-free) for a party mocktail that's kid-friendly, too. Don't discard the watermelon-cucumber pulp; you can whisk it into a salad vinaigrette with oil and vinegar. For fun, freeze watermelon balls and use as ice cubes in your drink. Or plop some sliced jalapeño or fresh mint leaves into an ice cube tray, add water, then freeze to create cool-looking ice cubes.

- Vegan
- Gluten-Free
- Nut-Free
- Dairy-Free
- No Added Sugar
- Kid-Friendly
- Great for Leftovers
- 15 Minutes or Less

TIME SAVER: Purchase precut watermelon.

TIP: For a spicy kick, blend in half a small jalapeño pepper with seeds rather than mint.

TIP: Watermelon rind is actually edible (and nutritious)! You can slice the rind into bite-sized pieces and toss into stir-fries or smoothies. Or, using a vegetable peeler, you can create "noodles" for a cool salad.

8 cups large watermelon cubes (2½ pounds)

1 cup thick slices unpeeled English cucumber, plus 4 thin slices for garnish

Juice of 1 lime (about 2 tablespoons)

¼ teaspoon sea salt

supercharger

12 fresh mint leaves (optional)

In a high-powered blender, combine the watermelon, thick cucumber slices, lime juice, salt, and mint leaves (if using), and blend on high until smooth, about 1 minute. Strain through a fine-mesh strainer and reserve the pulp for use in another recipe. Pour into glasses, garnish with the thin cucumber slices, and serve.

PER SERVING: Calories 60; Total Fat 0 g (Sat Fat 0 g); Protein 1 g; Carb 16 g; Fiber <1 g; Cholesterol 0 mg; Sodium 150 mg; Total Sugar 13 g (Added Sugar 0 g)

SERVINGS: 4

SERVING SIZE: 1 cup

PREP TIME: 5 minutes

COOK TIME: 0 minutes

EXCELLENT SOURCE OF: vitamin A, vitamin C

supercharger

Fresh mint supercharges this recipe even more by providing vitamin A and antioxidants.

triple berry lime smoothie

● Vegetarian
● Gluten-Free
● No Added Sugar
(without honey)
● Kid-Friendly
● 15 Minutes or Less

TIP: If using frozen mixed berries, add 1 cup of milk or milk alternative for ease in blending. (Adding the milk will make 3 servings instead of 2.)

SERVINGS: 2

SERVING SIZE: about 1⅓ cups each

PREP TIME: 8 minutes (plus banana freezing time)

COOK TIME: 0 minutes

EXCELLENT SOURCE OF: fiber, vitamin C, riboflavin, vitamin B$_6$, vitamin B$_{12}$, selenium

GOOD SOURCE OF: calcium, pantothenic acid, phosphorus

This gorgeous fuchsia smoothie is as beautiful to look at as it is good for you. It's the perfect balance of tart and sweet to awaken your taste buds, and is an excellent source of protein and fiber for staying power, along with mood-boosting nutrients like vitamin C, vitamin B$_6$, and selenium. You can choose your favorite three berries in the amounts you prefer.

1 ripe medium banana, peeled, broken into 4 pieces, and frozen

2 cups mixed fresh berries, such as blueberries, raspberries, and sliced strawberries

2 tablespoons fruit-sweetened seedless raspberry fruit spread or honey

½ teaspoon grated lime zest (from about ½ lime)

Juice of 2 limes (about ¼ cup)

1 cup low-fat (1% or 2%) plain Greek yogurt or Greek-style plant-based yogurt of choice

supercharger

2 teaspoons ground flaxseed (optional)

Combine the frozen banana, berries, fruit spread, lime zest, lime juice, yogurt, and flaxseed (if using) in a high-powered blender. Process on high until smooth and creamy, about 1½ minutes.

Pour into 2 chilled glasses and enjoy immediately!

PER SERVING: Calories 220; Total Fat 1 g (Sat Fat 0 g); Protein 13 g; Carb 42 g; Fiber 10 g; Cholesterol 5 mg; Sodium 40 mg; Total Sugar 21 g (Added Sugar 0g)

supercharger

Flaxseed supercharges this recipe even more by providing fiber, healthy fats, thiamin, and magnesium.

cinnamon pumpkin seed milk

Homemade nut or seed milk adds richness and flavor to breakfasts and can be used anywhere you'd use dairy milk, including in oatmeal, in a baking recipe, to enrich a soup, or simply enjoyed as is for an afternoon pick-me-up. If the idea of making your own seed milk sounds daunting, rest assured that the whole process takes less than 10 minutes. If you don't have a nut milk bag or cheesecloth, you can strain the pumpkin seed milk mixture three times directly through a clean fine-mesh strainer, using a flexible silicone spatula to help gently press the mixture through the strainer. Reserve the solids to use in smoothies or stir into oatmeal. If you choose to supercharge this recipe, the carrot adds a slight hint of natural sweetness.

● Vegan
● Gluten-Free
● Nut-Free
● Dairy-Free
● No Added Sugar
● Kid-Friendly
● 15 Minutes or Less

SERVINGS: 4

SERVING SIZE: about 1 cup

PREP TIME: 8 minutes

COOK TIME: 0 minutes

GOOD SOURCE OF: fiber, magnesium, zinc, copper

1 cup unsalted raw pumpkin seeds

4 cups cold filtered water

2 teaspoons unrefined (virgin) coconut oil

½ teaspoon pure vanilla extract (optional)

½ teaspoon ground cinnamon

¼ teaspoon sea salt

supercharger

½ medium carrot, peeled (optional)

Place a fine-mesh strainer over a large bowl, line with a nut milk bag or several layers of cheesecloth, and set aside.

Combine the pumpkin seeds, water, coconut oil, vanilla, cinnamon, salt, and carrot (if using) in a high-powered blender. Process on high until very smooth, about 3 minutes. Pour the resulting mixture into the nut milk bag or through the lined mesh strainer. Discard or reserve the solids for later use in a soup or smoothie.

Serve or use immediately, or transfer to a covered glass jar and refrigerate for up to 5 days. Shake or stir well before serving.

PER SERVING: Calories 90; Total Fat 5 g (Sat Fat 2.5 g); Protein 3 g; Carb 9 g; Fiber 3 g; Cholesterol 0 mg; Sodium 150 mg; Total Sugar 2 g (Added Sugar 0 g)

supercharger

Carrot supercharges this recipe even more by providing fiber, vitamin A, and vitamin K.

soups & stews

shiitake & herb broth in a hurry

Shiitakes lend an umami flavor to this savory broth that's so easy to make. It offers a boatload of B vitamins to help keep you energized, too. Zipping open a can of soup is easier, but it's never as good as homemade. Plan to enjoy this nourishing, immune-supporting broth regularly—and go ahead and double it! It's great for an appetizer, side, or snack. Serve with brown rice ramen noodles or wontons and top with sliced scallions to transform it into a hearty entrée-sized bowl of goodness.

6 cups water

2 large garlic cloves, peeled and smashed

1½ cups packed sliced fresh shiitake caps or maitake mushrooms (4.5 ounces)

1 tablespoon white miso paste

⅓ cup packed roughly chopped fresh cilantro, divided

¾ teaspoon sea salt, or to taste

½ teaspoon freshly ground black pepper, or to taste

supercharger

1-inch piece fresh ginger, peeled and thinly sliced (1 tablespoon) (optional)

- Vegan
- Gluten-Free
- Nut-Free
- Dairy-Free
- No Added Sugar
- Great for Leftovers
- Smart Freezer Meal
- 30 Minutes or Less

TIP: If you're not a fan of cilantro, substitute 1 scallion, green and white parts, thinly sliced.

SERVINGS: 4

SERVING SIZE: about 1 cup

PREP TIME: 8 minutes

COOK TIME: 17 minutes

EXCELLENT SOURCE OF: riboflavin, niacin, vitamin B₆, pantothenic acid, zinc, selenium, copper, manganese

GOOD SOURCE OF: fiber, potassium, thiamin, folate, phosphorus, magnesium

Place the water, garlic, and ginger (if using) in a stockpot or large saucepan set over high heat and bring to a boil. Add the mushrooms and return to a boil. Reduce heat to medium-high and cook at a gentle boil until the broth is richly fragrant, about 12 minutes. Discard the garlic and, ginger (if using). Turn off the heat and stir in the miso paste, ¼ cup of the cilantro, the salt, and the pepper. Taste to adjust for seasoning.

Pour into mugs or bowls, top with the remaining cilantro, and serve. Store broth in a large sealable container in the fridge for up to 1 week or in the freezer for up to 2 months.

PER SERVING: Calories 110; Total Fat 0.5 g (Sat Fat 0 g); Protein 5 g; Carb 27 g; Fiber 4 g; Cholesterol 0 mg; Sodium 610 mg; Total Sugar 2 g (Added Sugar 0 g)

supercharger

Fresh ginger supercharges this recipe even more by providing antioxidants that may prevent stress and disease.

sweet potato, tomato & turmeric soup

● Vegetarian
● Gluten-Free
● Nut-Free
● Great for Leftovers
● Smart Freezer Meal

TIP: Leave the sweet potato peel on for more fiber.

TIP: Black pepper unleashes the health benefits of turmeric by increasing its absorption.

SERVINGS: 8

SERVING SIZE: 1 cup

PREP TIME: 15 minutes

COOK TIME: 35 minutes

EXCELLENT SOURCE OF: fiber, iron, potassium, vitamin A, vitamin C, vitamin E, riboflavin, niacin, vitamin B$_6$, pantothenic acid, copper, manganese

GOOD SOURCE OF: vitamin K, thiamin, folate, phosphorus, magnesium, zinc

A serving of this velvety, warming bowl of comfort will make you feel happier at first sight, livelier at first smell, and healthier at first sip. It's health-protective thanks in part to antioxidants—crushed tomatoes provide lycopene and the sweet potato offers beta-carotene. The turmeric gives it potential anti-inflammatory properties, too. There's one more cool thing (literally!) about this soup: on warm days, you can serve it chilled, like gazpacho. This big batch keeps well in the fridge for days.

3 tablespoons unsalted butter

1 small yellow onion, sliced

1 large (14-ounce) sweet potato, peeled and finely chopped

2 teaspoons fresh grated turmeric or ¾ teaspoon ground turmeric

1 teaspoon sea salt, or to taste

¾ teaspoon freshly ground black pepper

1 (28-ounce) can crushed tomatoes (with juices)

1 (32-ounce) carton low-sodium vegetable broth

1 tablespoon red wine vinegar

2 teaspoons honey or coconut nectar

Handful of fresh cilantro leaves

supercharger

1 tablespoon mixed black and white sesame seeds (optional)

Heat the butter in a Dutch oven or large saucepan over medium-high heat. Once the butter melts, add the onion, sweet potato, turmeric, salt, and pepper and cook, stirring occasionally, until the onion is softened, about 5 minutes. Add the canned tomatoes with their juices and the broth and bring to a boil over high heat. Reduce heat to medium-low and simmer uncovered until the sweet potato can be easily mashed with a fork, about 22 minutes, stirring occasionally.

Working carefully, in a blender (or with an immersion wand blender), puree the soup in batches. Return pureed soup to the Dutch oven over medium-low heat, stir in the vinegar and honey, and cook just until heated through. Taste to adjust for seasoning.

To serve, ladle the soup into bowls and top with the cilantro and sesame seeds (if using).

The soup will keep well in an airtight container in the fridge for up to 4 days, or in the freezer for up to 3 months.

PER SERVING:
Calories 270; Total Fat 9 g (Sat Fat 5 g); Protein 5 g; Carb 44 g; Fiber 8 g; Cholesterol 25 mg; Sodium 790 mg; Total Sugar 19 g (Added Sugar 3 g)

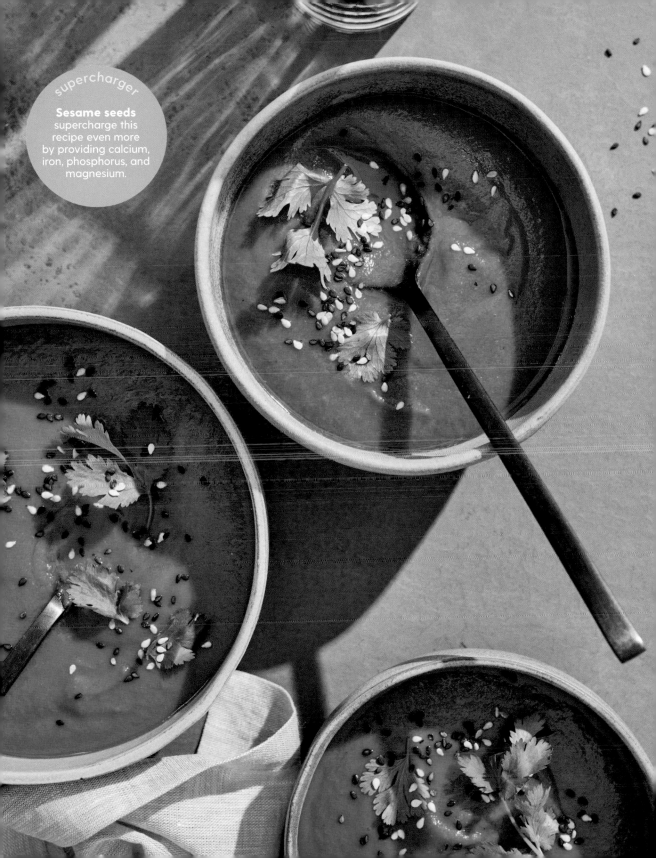

supercharger

Sesame seeds supercharge this recipe even more by providing calcium, iron, phosphorus, and magnesium.

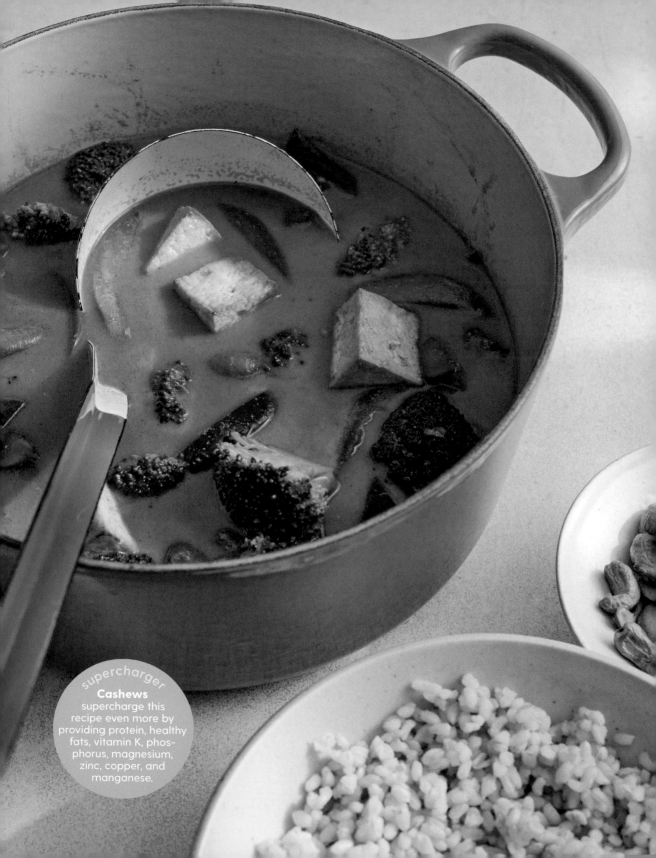

supercharger

Cashews supercharge this recipe even more by providing protein, healthy fats, vitamin K, phosphorus, magnesium, zinc, copper, and manganese.

one-pot thai red curry

Have you gotten all of your vitamins and minerals today? If not, this lightened-up tofu and veggie curry can help. It's an excellent source of 17 vitamins and minerals! But more important to your taste buds, it's absolutely luxurious tasting. And don't be intimidated by the ingredient list; once you get the items prepped and lined up, this curry is a relatively simple one-pot fix that counts as a complete meal. The more you make it, the easier it becomes. Plus, it stores well in the fridge or freezer for later.

- Vegan
- One-Dish Meal
- Gluten-Free (if using certified gluten-free tofu and certified gluten-free red curry paste)
- Dairy-Free
- Great for Leftovers
- Smart Freezer Meal

TIME SAVER: Use microwavable brown rice, ready in 3 minutes (or less!).

TIP: If you're not a fan of spicy food, this mild Thai dish is for you. But if you prefer spice, simply add sriracha, chili garlic sauce, or crushed red pepper flakes to taste before serving.

SERVINGS: 6

SERVING SIZE: 1 rounded cup curry + ¾ cup rice

PREP TIME: 25 minutes

COOK TIME: 20 minutes

EXCELLENT SOURCE OF: fiber, calcium, iron, vitamin A, vitamin C, vitamin K, thiamin, riboflavin, niacin, vitamin B$_6$, folate, pantothenic acid, phosphorus, magnesium, zinc, selenium, copper, manganese

GOOD SOURCE OF: potassium

2 tablespoons avocado oil or sunflower oil

1 (15.5- or 16-ounce) package extra-firm tofu, squeezed of excess liquid, cut into 1-inch cubes

1 small or ½ large yellow onion, diced

2 large red bell peppers, thinly sliced

3 tablespoons red curry paste

4 large garlic cloves, minced

2 teaspoons fresh grated ginger

1½ teaspoons sea salt

1⅔ cups cold water

1 tablespoon organic cornstarch

1 (13.5-ounce) can light coconut milk

¼ cup unsalted, unsweetened cashew butter or almond butter

1 tablespoon maple syrup

3 cups packed small broccoli florets or mixture of broccoli florets and snap peas

Juice of 1 lime (about 2 tablespoons)

4½ cups steamed brown rice, for serving

½ cup packed fresh cilantro leaves with tender stems

supercharger

½ cup salted roasted cashews, roughly chopped (optional)

In an extra-large saucepan or a Dutch oven, heat the oil over medium-high heat. When it shimmers, add the tofu and onion and cook, stirring occasionally, until the tofu begins to lightly brown and the onion is softened, about 8 minutes. (If the tofu sticks too much to your pan, you can drizzle in a little more oil.) Add the bell peppers and cook, stirring occasionally, until heated through, about 2 minutes. Add the curry paste, garlic, ginger, and salt and cook, stirring occasionally, until fragrant, about 2 minutes.

(recipe continues)

Whisk together the water and cornstarch in a small bowl, then add to the saucepan along with the coconut milk, nut butter, maple syrup, and broccoli and bring to a boil over high heat. Then reduce heat to medium and simmer, stirring occasionally, until the broccoli is crisp-tender and bright green, about 3 minutes. Stir in the lime juice and taste to adjust for seasoning.

Divide steamed rice among bowls, ladle in the curry, and sprinkle with the cashews (if using) and cilantro.

The curry keeps well in an airtight container in the fridge for up to 4 days, or properly stored in the freezer for about 4 months. Freeze any extras in pre-portioned containers for a healthy meal reheated in minutes.

PER SERVING: Calories 480; Total Fat 22 g (Sat Fat 6 g); Protein 21 g; Carb 53 g; Fiber 8 g; Cholesterol 0 mg; Sodium 800 mg; Total Sugar 8 g (Added Sugar 2 g)

garlic, lentil & carrot soup

If you think a cup of soup isn't filling, you haven't met Garlic, Lentil, and Carrot Soup! So, let me introduce you to this bowl of plant-based goodness. It's a "wow" for protein and fiber. The Swiss chard not only supercharges the nutrition but also boosts the taste and visual appeal. Make extra and store in individual containers in the freezer for a nourishing meal in minutes. It doesn't get more satisfying than slurping up this soup. Serve along with a toasty baguette.

- Vegan (without Parmesan cheese topping)
- Gluten-Free
- Nut-Free
- Dairy-Free (without Parmesan cheese topping)
- No Added Sugar
- Great for Leftovers
- Smart Freezer Meal

3 tablespoons extra-virgin olive oil

1 medium yellow onion, finely diced

2 large carrots, scrubbed or peeled, finely chopped (1 cup)

1 large (8-ounce) russet potato, scrubbed, unpeeled, and diced small

5 large garlic cloves, minced

½ teaspoon ground coriander

1½ teaspoons sea salt

1 teaspoon freshly ground black pepper

6 cups low-sodium vegetable broth

2 (15-ounce) cans no-salt-added lentils, drained

Juice of 1 lemon (about 3 tablespoons)

Suggested Toppings: grated Parmesan cheese, chopped fresh flat-leaf parsley, crushed red pepper flakes

supercharger

3 cups packed roughly chopped Swiss chard, ribs and thick stems removed (optional)

TIME SAVER: Use jarred or frozen minced garlic. Typically, ½ teaspoon minced garlic from a jar equals one fresh garlic clove, minced.

SERVINGS: 10

SERVING SIZE: 1 cup

PREP TIME: 20 minutes

COOK TIME: 30 minutes

EXCELLENT SOURCE OF: fiber, iron, vitamin A, folate, copper, manganese

GOOD SOURCE OF: potassium, thiamin, vitamin B$_6$, pantothenic acid, phosphorus, magnesium, zinc

Heat the oil in a Dutch oven or stockpot over medium heat. When the oil shimmers, add the onion, carrots, potato, garlic, coriander, salt, and pepper and cook, stirring occasionally, until the onion is softened, about 8 minutes. Add the broth and bring to a boil over high heat. Add the lentils, reduce heat to medium, and simmer uncovered until all vegetables are tender, about 15 minutes.

Add the Swiss chard, if using, and cook until wilted, about 2 minutes. Add the lemon juice. Taste to adjust for seasoning. Transfer to bowls, add toppings, if desired, and serve.

The soup keeps well in an airtight container in the fridge for 4 days or in the freezer for up to 3 months.

PER SERVING: Calories 170; Total Fat 4.5 g (Sat Fat 0.5 g); Protein 9 g; Carb 26 g; Fiber 8 g; Cholesterol 0 mg; Sodium 640 mg; Total Sugar 4 g (Added Sugar 0 g)

supercharger

Swiss chard supercharges this recipe even more by providing vitamin A, vitamin C, and vitamin K.

cauliflower & black bean chili

- Vegan
- One-Dish Meal
- Gluten-Free
- Nut-Free
- Dairy-Free
- No Added Sugar
- Kid-Friendly
- Great for Leftovers
- Smart Freezer Meal

TIME SAVERS: Triple or quadruple the Spice Mixture recipe. Save and label it "Cauliflower and Black Bean Chili Spice Mixture" for later. Simply use 3 tablespoons of the mixture every time you make this recipe.

Buy precut cauliflower florets.

SERVINGS: 8

SERVING SIZE: 1½ cups

PREP TIME: 25 minutes

COOK TIME: 30 minutes

EXCELLENT SOURCE OF: fiber, iron, potassium, vitamin A, vitamin C, vitamin K, thiamin, riboflavin, vitamin B$_6$, folate, pantothenic acid, magnesium, copper, manganese

GOOD SOURCE OF: calcium, vitamin E, niacin, phosphorus, zinc

Even meat eaters will embrace this full-flavored, fiber-rich vegan chili. It takes some inspiration from Mexican cuisine to give it extra scrumptiousness. While it's perfect as is, you can play with it by adding whatever toppings you like. It'll be a hit if you make a chili "bar" by setting out various garnishes, such as lime wedges, fresh cilantro, diced red onion, sliced radishes, and shredded Cheddar or plant-based cheese. It can be paired with some warm corn tortillas or tortilla chips for a fun meal, too.

spice mixture

2 teaspoons chili powder

2 teaspoons ground coriander

1½ teaspoons dried oregano

1 teaspoon sea salt

1 teaspoon freshly ground black pepper

1 teaspoon paprika

½ teaspoon ground cumin or cinnamon

chili

¼ cup avocado oil or extra-virgin olive oil

1 large sweet onion, diced

4 large garlic cloves, minced

2 tablespoons no-salt-added tomato paste

1 medium head cauliflower, cut into small florets (about 6 cups florets)

1 large green bell pepper, diced

2 (15-ounce) cans low-sodium black beans, drained

1 (28-ounce) can crushed tomatoes

2½ cups low-sodium vegetable broth

supercharger

2 avocados, cubed (optional)

Stir together all of the spice mixture ingredients in a small bowl and set aside.

Heat the oil in a Dutch oven or stockpot over medium-high heat. When it shimmers, carefully add the onion and cook, stirring occasionally, until softened, about 5 minutes. Add the garlic and cook while stirring until fragrant, about 1 minute. Add the tomato paste and spice mixture and cook while stirring until fragrant, about 1 minute.

Add the cauliflower, bell pepper, beans, crushed tomatoes, and broth, increase heat to high, and bring to a boil. Then reduce heat to medium and simmer uncovered until the chili reaches your desired flavor depth and consistency, at least 20 minutes. (Note: After cooking, the chili will thicken a bit more as it stands.) Taste to adjust for seasoning. If you find the flavor is too intense, add more broth.

To serve, ladle the chili into bowls and top with the avocado, if using. Garnish with your favorite fixings, such as lime wedges, fresh cilantro, diced onion, or sliced radishes.

Chili will last well in an airtight container in the fridge for up to 4 days, or properly stored in the freezer for about 4 months. Freeze any extras in pre-portioned containers for a nourishing meal reheated in minutes.

PER SERVING: Calories 240; Total Fat 8 g (Sat Fat 1 g); Protein 10 g; Carb 36 g; Fiber 15 g; Cholesterol 0 mg; Sodium 550 mg; Total Sugar 11 g (Added Sugar 0 g)

supercharger
Avocado supercharges this recipe even more by providing fiber, healthy fats, vitamin C, vitamin K, vitamin B_6, folate, potassium, and antioxidants.

miso soup
with greens & tofu

- Vegan
- Gluten-Free
- Nut-Free
- Dairy-Free
- No Added Sugar
- Great for Leftovers
- Smart Freezer Meal
- 30 Minutes or Less

TIP: For an entrée version, double the serving size to 2½ cups and add in edamame or shrimp for bonus high-quality protein.

SERVINGS: 8

SERVING SIZE: 1¼ cups

PREP TIME: 8 minutes

COOK TIME: 12 minutes

EXCELLENT SOURCE OF: calcium, vitamin A, vitamin K, manganese

GOOD SOURCE OF: iron, selenium, copper

Miso is fermented soybean paste. It adds flavor pow to anything you pair it with. Plus the probiotics in miso may help strengthen your gut flora, in turn boosting your immunity. One of the most popular ways to use it is in miso soup, a traditional Japanese dish. This green veggie-filled version is so simple to make. Its trio of tofu, leafy greens, and seaweed makes the soup an excellent source of calcium, which supports mood and sleep.

2 (32-ounce) cartons low-sodium vegetable broth

¼ teaspoon sea salt

⅓ cup white miso paste

8 ounces firm or soft tofu (with calcium), squeezed of excess liquid, cubed (1½ cups)

2 cups packed fresh baby spinach

2 cups packed chopped green Swiss chard or kale, stems removed

3 scallions, green and white parts, thinly sliced

2 sheets dried nori seaweed, chopped into wedges

supercharger

1 red hot chili pepper, extra-thinly sliced crosswise (optional)

Place the broth and salt in a stockpot or large saucepan and bring to a gentle simmer over medium heat.

Place the miso paste in a small bowl, ladle ⅓ cup of the simmering broth over the paste, and whisk to make a slurry. Set aside.

Add the tofu, spinach, Swiss chard, and scallions to the broth and cook until the tofu is heated through, about 3 minutes. Stir in the miso slurry, chopped nori, and hot chili pepper (if using) to combine. Taste to adjust for seasoning, adding a little more miso or a few drops of tamari or soy sauce if needed, and serve warm.

Once cooled, the soup can be stored in an airtight container in the fridge for up to 3 days, or pour into freezer-safe containers and freeze for up to 6 months. Store in pre-portioned containers for a quick heat-and-serve soup.

PER SERVING: Calories 80; Total Fat 3 g (Sat Fat 0 g); Protein 7 g; Carb 8 g; Fiber 2 g; Cholesterol 0 mg; Sodium 700 mg; Total Sugar 5 g (Added Sugar 0 g)

supercharger
Hot chili pepper supercharges this recipe even more by providing capsaicin, which may help dampen inflammation and promote heart health.

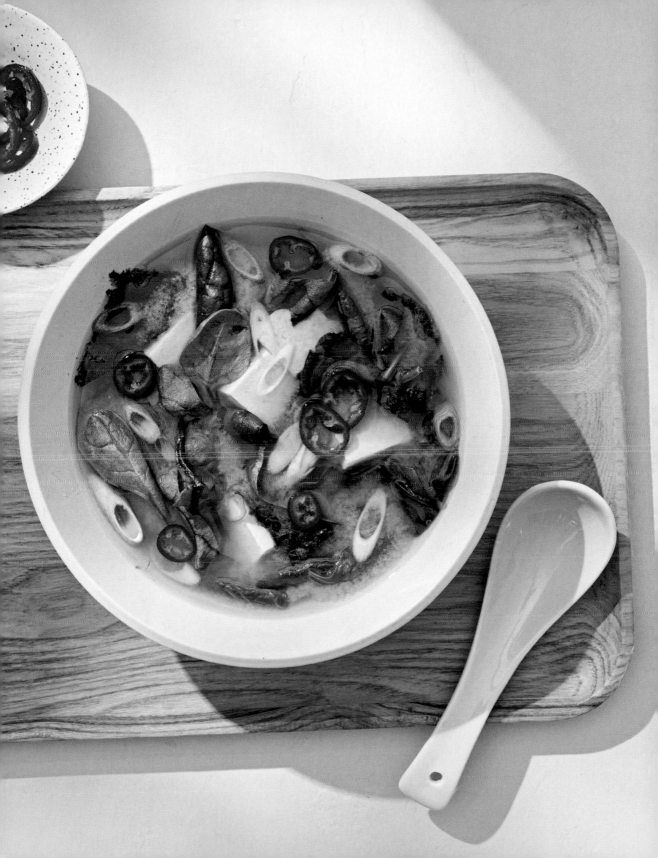

salads
&
sides

fig & grapefruit salad
with pomegranate rosemary vinaigrette

supercharger

Pomegranate arils supercharge this recipe even more by providing fiber, vitamin C, vitamin K, and antioxidants.

Fruits and vegetables team up in this salad that offers just the right balance of sweet and savory. The peppery, slightly bitter arugula balances beautifully with the sweet figs and tart grapefruit, but feel free to use any greens you have on hand. My favorite part is the homemade ruby-red dressing, which brings an aromatic, fruit-filled, fall-inspired touch. When pomegranate is in season, supercharge this salad with antioxidant-rich arils for a juicy crunch. Enjoy as a side dish or add your favorite protein to make it a full meal!

- Vegetarian (or vegan if using coconut nectar in dressing)
- Gluten-Free
- Nut-Free
- Dairy-Free
- Kid-Friendly
- Great for Leftovers (vinaigrette only)
- 15 Minutes or Less

TIME SAVER: Use bottled organic or natural poppyseed or honey mustard dressing.

TIP: A nice semihard sheep's milk cheese, aged goat cheese, or aged nut cheese is a tasty addition to this salad, if you want bonus indulgence.

SERVINGS: 4

SERVING SIZE: 1½ cups

PREP TIME: 15 minutes

COOK TIME: 0 minutes

EXCELLENT SOURCE OF: vitamin A, vitamin C, vitamin K

GOOD SOURCE OF: fiber, vitamin B$_6$, pantothenic acid, copper, manganese

rosemary pomegranate vinaigrette

½ cup 100% pomegranate juice

Juice of 1 small lemon (about 2 tablespoons)

1 tablespoon honey or coconut nectar

2 teaspoons minced fresh rosemary

1 teaspoon Dijon mustard

⅓ cup extra-virgin olive oil

¼ teaspoon sea salt

salad

1 small shallot, thinly sliced

3 cups packed fresh baby arugula leaves (3 ounces)

8 medium or 6 large fresh black Mission or other figs, quartered lengthwise

½ teaspoon freshly ground black pepper

1 medium ruby red or pink grapefruit, cut into segments or thin wedges

supercharger

¼ cup pomegranate arils (optional)

Make the vinaigrette: Whisk all of the ingredients for the vinaigrette in a small bowl or shake in a jar and set aside. Note: You'll have more dressing than needed for this salad. (Makes 1 cup.)

Make the salad: Combine ⅓ cup of the vinaigrette and the shallot in a large mixing bowl. (Reserve the remaining dressing for another use.) Add the arugula, figs, and pepper and toss to coat. Add the grapefruit and toss gently to combine. Transfer to a serving dish or salad plates. Sprinkle with the pomegranate arils, if using. Enjoy immediately.

Dressing keeps well in an airtight container in the fridge for up to 1 week.

PER SERVING (WITH ⅓ CUP VINAIGRETTE, TOTAL): Calories 170; Total Fat 7 g (Sat Fat 1 g); Protein 2 g; Carb 30 g; Fiber 5 g; Cholesterol 0 mg; Sodium 160 mg; Total Sugar 23 g (Added Sugar 1 g)

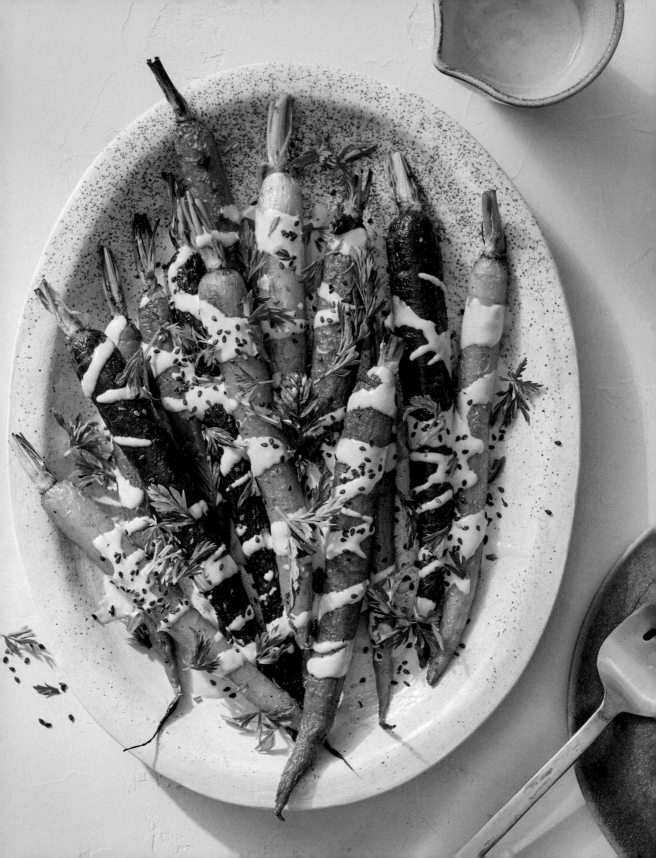

tricolor roasted carrots
with cardamom
tahini sauce

Sure, you can nibble on some raw baby carrots. But if you want to appreciate carrots in a whole new way, this roasted side dish is a dazzler. Using tricolor carrots and leaving on part of the tops provides intrigue. And do be sure to look for carrots that still have their leafy tops; you'll want them to supercharge this recipe. What if you want a grain side, too? Go for it by serving these roasted carrots with sauce on top of a bed of barley, farro, freekeh, or bulgur.

- Vegan
- Gluten-Free
- Nut-Free
- Dairy-Free
- No Added Sugar
- Kid-Friendly
- Great for Leftovers

TIME SAVERS: Use a bottled organic or natural creamy tahini dressing. Use packaged baby carrots and reduce cooking time.

TIP: If you have extra carrot tops, consider using them to make carrot top pesto or chimichurri—or use as some of the herbs in the Fresh Herb Hummus (page 131).

SERVINGS: 4

SERVING SIZE: 4 carrots

PREP TIME: 12 minutes

COOK TIME: 30 minutes

EXCELLENT SOURCE OF: fiber, vitamin A, vitamin C, vitamin K, thiamin, vitamin B$_6$, copper

GOOD SOURCE OF: potassium, vitamin E, riboflavin, niacin, folate, pantothenic acid, phosphorus, manganese

roasted carrots

16 medium (about 8-inch) tricolor carrots with leafy tops (about 2 pounds)

2 tablespoons extra-virgin olive oil

½ teaspoon sea salt

½ teaspoon freshly ground black pepper

1½ teaspoons toasted sesame seeds (optional)

cardamom tahini sauce

¼ cup tahini

Juice of 1 lemon (about 3 tablespoons)

3 tablespoons unsweetened green tea or water

¼ teaspoon ground cumin

¼ teaspoon ground cardamom

¼ teaspoon sea salt

1 large garlic clove, minced (optional)

supercharger

3 tablespoons roughly chopped leafy carrot tops (optional)

Preheat the oven to 425°F.

Scrub the carrots (do not peel). Pat dry. Trim carrot tops to about 1½ inches in length. If using, roughly chop and reserve 3 tablespoons of the leafy carrot tops for the supercharger.

Set the carrots on a rimmed baking sheet, drizzle with the olive oil, and toss to coat. Sprinkle with the salt and pepper and toss to coat. Roast until caramelized and just tender, about 22 to 25 minutes, shaking the baking sheet to rotate carrots halfway through roasting.

(recipe continues)

supercharger

Carrot tops
supercharge this
recipe even more by
providing fiber,
potassium, vitamin A,
vitamin C,
and antioxidants.

Meanwhile, prepare the sauce: Whisk together all the sauce ingredients in a small bowl until smooth and set aside. Note: You'll have more dressing than needed for this salad. (Makes about ⅔ cup.)

Transfer the carrots to a serving platter (or serve from the baking sheet) and drizzle with ⅓ cup of the tahini sauce. (Reserve the remaining sauce for another use.) If using, sprinkle with the sesame seeds and carrot tops to serve.

Roasted carrots keep well in an airtight container in the refrigerator for up to 4 days. Sauce keeps well in an airtight container in the fridge for up to 1 week.

PER SERVING (with ⅓ cup dressing, total): Calories 200; Total Fat 11 g (Sat Fat 1.5 g); Protein 4 g; Carb 24 g; Fiber 7 g; Cholesterol 0 mg; Sodium 520 mg; Total Sugar 11 g (Added Sugar 0 g)

cashew chinese salad
with miso mustard dressing

This salad is packed with an array of nutrient-dense veggies like leafy greens, red cabbage, and carrots. Immunity-boosting mandarin oranges add a juicy sweetness and pair perfectly with salty and crunchy cashews. But the real secret here is the Miso Mustard Dressing, which gives this recipe an umami kick. To make this salad a meal, supercharge it with store-bought sesame ginger baked tofu.

- Vegan
- Gluten-Free
- Dairy-Free
- Great for Leftovers (dressing only)
- 30 Minutes or Less

TIME SAVER: Use bottled organic or natural sesame ginger dressing.

SERVINGS: 4

SERVING SIZE: about 2 cups

PREP TIME: 20 minutes

COOK TIME: 0 minutes

EXCELLENT SOURCE OF: vitamin A, vitamin C, vitamin K, copper, manganese

GOOD SOURCE OF: fiber, iron, thiamin, vitamin B$_6$, phosphorus, magnesium, zinc

miso mustard dressing

¼ cup rice vinegar

2 tablespoons white miso paste

2 tablespoons Dijon mustard

2 tablespoons maple syrup

½ cup avocado oil or sunflower oil

¼ teaspoon sea salt

¼ teaspoon freshly ground black pepper

salad

1 (5-ounce) package mixed baby salad greens

¾ cup fresh or drained canned mandarin orange segments

⅔ cup extra-thinly sliced red cabbage

2 scallions, green and white parts, thinly sliced

⅓ cup grated carrot (from 1 medium carrot)

¼ teaspoon sea salt

½ cup salted roasted cashews

½ cup fresh cilantro leaves with tender stems

supercharger

6 to 8 ounces sesame ginger baked tofu (store-bought), cubed (optional)

Make the dressing: Whisk all of the ingredients for the dressing in a medium bowl or shake in a jar and set aside. Note: You'll have more dressing than needed for this salad. (Makes 1 cup plus 2 tablespoons.)

Make the salad: Add the salad greens, mandarin oranges, cabbage, scallions, carrot, and salt to a large mixing bowl and toss to combine. Add ⅓ cup of the dressing and toss to coat. (Reserve remaining dressing for another use.) Add the cashews and toss to combine. Transfer salad to plates. Top with tofu (if using), and cilantro. Enjoy immediately. Dressing will last in an airtight container, such as a mason jar, in the refrigerator for up to 1 week.

PER SERVING (with ⅓ cup dressing): Calories 220; Total Fat 16 g (Sat Fat 2.5 g); Protein 5 g; Carb 17 g; Fiber 3 g; Cholesterol 0 mg; Sodium 390 mg; Total Sugar 9 g (Added Sugar 2 g)

supercharger

Tofu supercharges this recipe even more by providing protein, calcium, and iron.

peach salad with lemony poppyseed dressing

When peaches are in season, this salad is what you need in your life. It showcases how well the juicy fruit pairs with seasonings and savory ingredients. The lemony poppyseed dressing adds fresh vibrancy and, of course, citrusy aroma. An ancient whole wheat grain, farro complements the salad by adding a chewy texture and nutty flavor. The Marcona almonds make it extra special. This is one of my favorite summer salads!

● Vegetarian
● Nut-Free (without almonds)
● Great for Leftovers (dressing only)
● 30 Minutes or Less

TIME SAVERS: Use 90-second microwavable farro or whole-grain mixture. Use bottled organic or natural poppyseed dressing.

SERVINGS: 6

SERVING SIZE: 1½ rounded cups

PREP TIME: 25 minutes (with precooked farro)

COOK TIME: 0 minutes

EXCELLENT SOURCE OF: fiber, vitamin A, vitamin K, copper

GOOD SOURCE OF: iron, vitamin C, vitamin E, folate, pantothenic acid, manganese

lemony poppyseed dressing

1 teaspoon grated lemon zest

Juice of 2 lemons (about ¼ cup plus 2 tablespoons)

½ cup plus 2 tablespoons extra-virgin olive oil

1½ tablespoons honey

1 tablespoon Dijon mustard

1 tablespoon poppy seeds

½ teaspoon sea salt

½ teaspoon freshly ground black pepper

salad

2 small (4-ounce) or 1 large (8-ounce) head butter (Bibb) lettuce, cored and roughly chopped

1 cup cooked farro, chilled

¼ teaspoon plus ⅛ teaspoon sea salt, divided

½ teaspoon freshly ground black pepper, divided

2 ripe yellow peaches, pitted and cut into wedges

1 large avocado, sliced

½ cup crumbled goat cheese

supercharger

⅓ cup Marcona almonds or pan-toasted slivered natural almonds (optional)

Make the dressing: Whisk all of the ingredients for the dressing in a medium bowl or shake in a jar and set aside. Note: You'll have more dressing than needed for this salad. (Makes 1 cup plus 3 tablespoons.)

Make the salad: Arrange the lettuce on a large serving platter.

In a small mixing bowl, combine the farro, 1½ tablespoons of the dressing, ⅛ teaspoon of the salt, and ¼ teaspoon of the pepper and stir to combine; scatter the farro mixture over the lettuce.

Arrange the peaches and avocado on the salad and drizzle with about ½ cup of the dressing, or to taste. (Reserve the remaining dressing for another use.) Sprinkle with the remaining ¼ teaspoon salt and ¼ teaspoon pepper, the goat cheese, and almonds (if using). Enjoy immediately. Dressing will last in an airtight container, such as a mason jar, in the refrigerator for up to 1 week.

PER SERVING (WITH HALF RECIPE DRESSING, TOTAL): Calories 270; Total Fat 18 g (Sat Fat 3.5 g); Protein 6 g; Carb 23 g; Fiber 5 g; Cholesterol <5 mg; Sodium 320 mg; Total Sugar 7 g (Added Sugar 2 g)

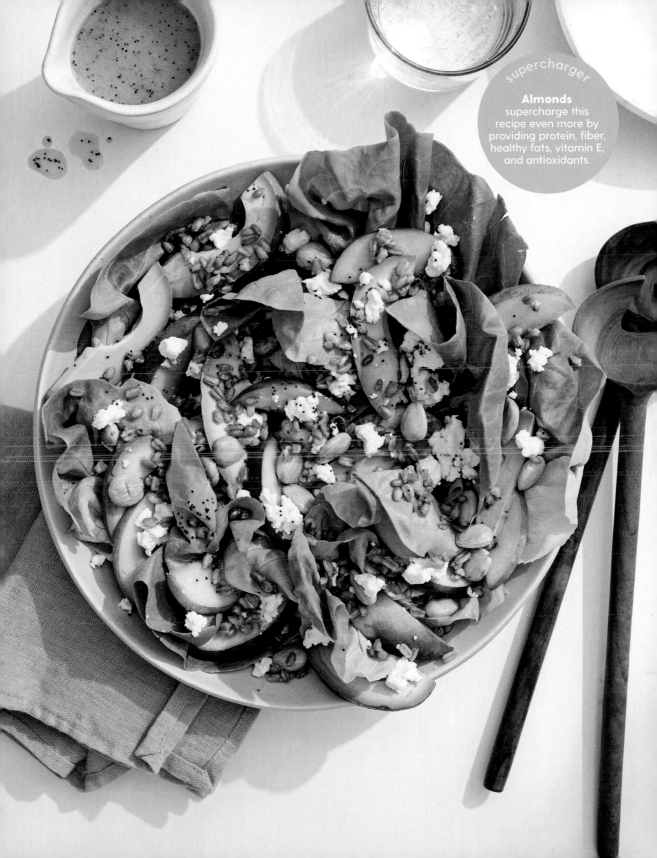

supercharger

Almonds supercharge this recipe even more by providing protein, fiber, healthy fats, vitamin E, and antioxidants.

kale, sweet potato & grape salad
with walnuts

- Vegetarian
- Gluten-Free
- Great for Leftovers
- 30 Minutes or Less

TIME SAVER: Purchase a bag of ready-to-use chopped kale.

TIP: I call this dressing my "Super Basic" because it works great on pretty much any salad. Double or triple the recipe to have more salad dressing on hand all week!

TIP: Bake an extra sweet potato to make the Avocado Sweet Potato Toast with a Fried Egg on page 107; it's a special way to start your day!

SERVINGS: 8 side salads (or 4 entrée salads)

SERVING SIZE: About 1½ cups for a side salad, or about 3 cups for a large salad

PREP TIME: 18 minutes

COOK TIME: 0 minutes (with prebaked sweet potato)

EXCELLENT SOURCE OF: calcium, vitamin A, vitamin C, vitamin K, folate, copper, manganese

GOOD SOURCE OF: fiber, vitamin B$_6$, magnesium

I love this salad for its taste, ease, and above all its versatility. It's the perfect salad to enjoy throughout the fall and winter, and it's great for entertaining. Winter vegetables like kale and sweet potatoes add a hearty touch and blend wonderfully with the crunchy fennel and sweet grapes. My favorite part? Pecorino cheese and walnuts offer just the right amount of flavor and healthy fats, so you'll finish feeling physically *and* mentally satisfied. While most salads are best eaten immediately, due to the heartiness of the kale and the lightness of the dressing, you can enjoy this salad as a leftover for a day or two—so why not double it!

super basic dressing

¼ cup extra-virgin olive oil

1 teaspoon grated lemon zest

Juice of 1 lemon (about 3 tablespoons)

2 teaspoons apple cider vinegar

2 teaspoons Dijon mustard

2 teaspoons maple syrup

1 medium garlic clove, minced

⅛ teaspoon sea salt

¼ teaspoon freshly ground black pepper

salad

2 bunches purple and green kale, chopped with stems and thick ribs removed (8 cups packed)

1 medium baked sweet potato (see page 187), chilled, peeled, cut into 1-inch cubes

1½ cups seedless red grapes, halved

½ cup walnut halves, roughly chopped

3 ounces pecorino cheese, thinly shaved, divided

supercharger

½ bulb fennel, cored and thinly sliced (optional)

Make the dressing: Whisk all of the ingredients for the dressing in a medium bowl or shake in a jar. Taste to adjust for seasoning and set aside. (Makes ⅔ cup dressing.)

Make the salad: In a large serving bowl, spoon 2 tablespoons of the dressing over the kale and "massage" together, gently squeezing and rubbing handfuls at a time until the kale is slightly less firm and more fragrant, about 1 minute. Add the sweet potato, grapes, fennel (if using), walnuts, and half of the pecorino to the bowl. Drizzle with the remaining dressing and gently toss just until all of the ingredients are evenly coated, being careful not to mash the sweet potato pieces. Taste to adjust for seasoning.

To serve, top with the remaining shaved pecorino. Serve at room temperature or chilled. Leftovers will keep well in the fridge, covered, for up to 2 days.

PER SERVING (as a side salad, with ⅔ cup dressing): Calories 210; Total Fat 14 g (Sat Fat 3.5 g); Protein 8 g; Carb 18 g; Fiber 3 g; Cholesterol 10 mg; Sodium 270 mg; Total Sugar 9 g (Added Sugar 1 g)

supercharger

Fennel
supercharges this recipe even more by providing fiber, potassium, and vitamin C.

how to bake sweet potatoes

Making baked sweet potatoes in the oven is so easy and brings out their natural flavor and sweetness.

Choose several medium sweet potatoes, uniform in size and shape. Preheat the oven to 425°F and line a baking sheet with parchment paper.

Wash, scrub, and dry each sweet potato thoroughly and transfer to the prepared baking sheet. Using a paring knife or fork, pierce each sweet potato in six places.

Transfer potatoes to the oven and bake until a knife or fork can easily be inserted into the thickest part, 40 to 45 minutes, rotating each half-way through the baking process to ensure even cooking. Remove from the oven and allow to cool for at least 1 hour.

For later use, store in an airtight container in the fridge for up to 3 days or freeze for up to 2 months.

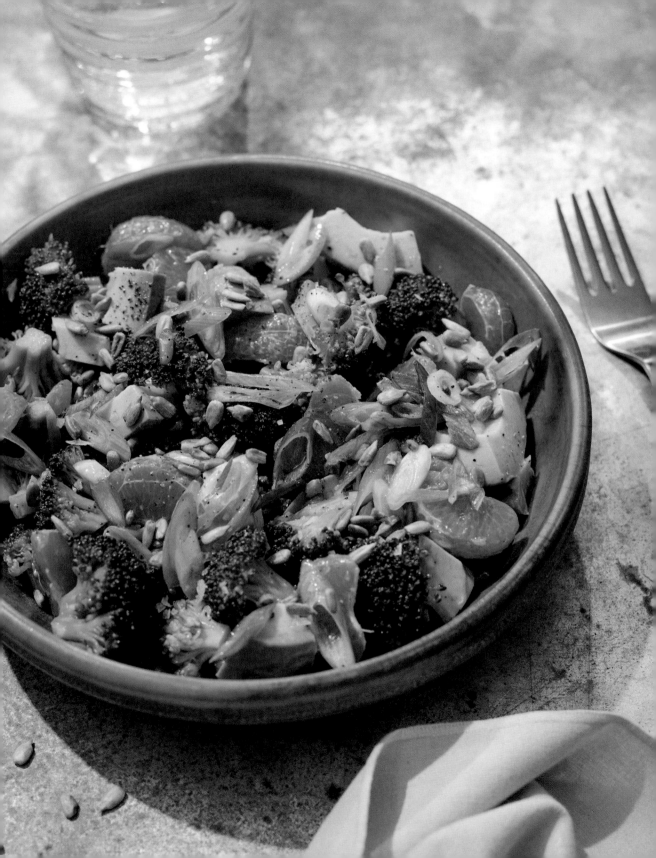

broccoli mandarin salad with ginger scallion dressing

This salad makes getting your veggies a tasty and gingery endeavor. You'll enjoy the pops of creamy avocado, sweet mandarin oranges, and crunchy sunflower seeds, but the broccoli is the star. The warm scallion dressing adds a bit of Asian flair with fresh ginger, thin scallions, and a dash of honey. An excellent source of mood-boosting nutrients like fiber, vitamin A, and vitamin C in this salad will make you feel as good as it tastes.

- Vegetarian
- Gluten-Free
- Nut-Free
- Dairy-Free
- Great for Leftovers (dressing only)
- 30 Minutes or Less

TIME SAVER: Purchase precut or frozen broccoli florets.

SERVINGS: 4

SERVING SIZE: 1½ cups

PREP TIME: 20 minutes

COOK TIME: 6 minutes

EXCELLENT SOURCE OF: vitamin A, vitamin C, vitamin K, folate, pantothenic acid

GOOD SOURCE OF: fiber, potassium, vitamin E, thiamin, riboflavin, vitamin B$_6$, phosphorus, selenium, copper, manganese

ginger scallion dressing

¾ cup avocado oil or sunflower oil

6 scallions, green and white parts, thinly sliced (about 1½ cups)

¼ cup rice vinegar

3 tablespoons fresh grated ginger

1 teaspoon honey or coconut nectar

½ teaspoon sea salt

½ teaspoon freshly ground black pepper

salad

1 pound small (about ¾-inch) broccoli florets (about 8 cups)

¾ cup fresh or drained canned mandarin orange segments

¼ teaspoon sea salt

½ teaspoon freshly ground black pepper

2 tablespoons salted roasted sunflower seeds

supercharger

1 large avocado, cubed (optional)

Make the dressing: Heat the oil in a large sauté pan over medium-high heat. Add the scallions and cook, stirring, until the oil is very fragrant, about 3 minutes. Remove from heat and carefully transfer the scallions and oil to a wide-mouthed glass jar or heatproof bowl. Shake with (or whisk in) the vinegar, ginger, honey, salt, and pepper. Taste to adjust for seasoning and set aside. Note: You'll have more dressing than needed for this salad. (Makes 1⅓ cups.)

Make the salad: Bring a large saucepan of salted water to a boil over high heat. Once boiling, add the broccoli and cook until bright green and just barely tender, about 2 minutes. Drain the broccoli through a large

(recipe continues)

supercharger
Avocado supercharges this recipe even more by providing fiber, healthy fats, potassium, vitamin C, vitamin K, vitamin B$_6$, folate, and antioxidants.

strainer and let stand in the strainer to fully drain and slightly cool, about 3 minutes.

Combine the broccoli and ⅓ cup of the dressing in a large salad bowl and stir to coat. (Reserve the remaining dressing for a later use.) Add the mandarin oranges, salt, pepper, and avocado (if using), and gently stir to just combine. Sprinkle with the sunflower seeds and serve chilled or at room temperature.

Dressed broccoli salad keeps well covered in the fridge for up to 2 days. Dressing will last in an airtight container, such as a mason jar, in the refrigerator for up to 1 week.

PER SERVING (with ⅓ cup dressing, total): Calories 180; Total Fat 13 g (Sat Fat 1.5 g); Protein 4 g; Carb 15 g; Fiber 4 g; Cholesterol 0 mg; Sodium 210 mg*; Total Sugar 7 g (Added Sugar 0 g)
* Sodium does not include salt added to water for broccoli prep.

mixed green, herb & olive salad

Call on this salad when your energy is low—it's packed with energy-boosting nutrients, and takes only 15 minutes to prepare. Simply toss a few handfuls of mixed baby salad greens with fresh herbs and top with pecorino cheese. Add in some walnuts, if you choose to supercharge it, for additional brain-boosting nutrients and crunch. The magic happens when this salad is dressed with the homemade vinaigrette that's loaded with green olives . . . like a big taste of Sicily. To make it a meal, couple the salad with protein like grilled fish or serve it with an omelet for an afternoon brunch.

- Vegetarian
- Gluten-Free
- Nut-Free (without walnuts)
- 15 Minutes or Less

TIME SAVER: Use bottled organic or natural red wine vinaigrette.

TIP: For a nuttier taste if you plan to use the supercharger, pan-toast the walnut halves in a dry skillet over medium heat until golden and fragrant, 3 to 5 minutes, then chop and fold into the recipe.

SERVINGS: 4

SERVING SIZE: 2 cups

PREP TIME: 15 minutes (including dressing prep)

COOK TIME: 0 minutes

EXCELLENT SOURCE OF: calcium, vitamin A, vitamin C, vitamin E, vitamin K

GOOD SOURCE OF: iron

green olive vinaigrette

3 tablespoons red wine vinegar

1 tablespoon honey

1 medium garlic clove, minced

½ cup extra-virgin olive oil

½ cup chopped pitted Castelvetrano or other green olives

¼ teaspoon sea salt

½ teaspoon freshly ground black pepper

salad

8 cups packed mixed baby salad greens (8 ounces)

1 cup mixed herbs, such as flat-leaf parsley, mint, and dill, chopped

2 ounces pecorino or Parmesan cheese, shaved

supercharger

⅔ cup walnut halves, raw or toasted, chopped (optional)

Make the dressing: Whisk all of the ingredients for the dressing in a medium bowl or shake in a jar and set aside. Note: You may have more dressing than needed for this salad. (Makes about 1 cup.)

Make the salad: Combine the salad greens, herbs, and walnuts (if using) in a large serving bowl. Spoon on about ⅔ cup of the dressing, or to taste, and gently toss to combine. Top with the shaved cheese and serve immediately. Serve remaining dressing on the side or reserve for later use. Dressing will last in an airtight container, such as a mason jar, in the refrigerator for up to 1 week.

PER SERVING (with ⅔ cup dressing, total): Calories 260; Total Fat 22 g (Sat Fat 6 g); Protein 7 g; Carb 12 g; Fiber 1 g; Cholesterol 15 mg; Sodium 520 mg; Total Sugar 6 g (Added Sugar 3 g)

supercharger

Walnuts
supercharge this recipe even more by providing protein, fiber, healthy fats, and antioxidants.

heirloom tomato & beet salad with ricotta

- Vegetarian
- Gluten-Free
- Nut-Free (without pine nuts)
- No Added Sugar
- Kid-Friendly
- 15 Minutes or Less

TIP: If you like to experiment with dairy offerings, this platter is also delightful prepared with quark or labneh in place of the ricotta cheese.

TIP: For a nutty flavor boost, toast the pine nuts in a dry skillet over medium heat, turning frequently, until golden in spots, 3 to 5 minutes.

SERVINGS: 4

SERVING SIZE: ¼ of platter

PREP TIME: 12 minutes

COOK TIME: 0 minutes

EXCELLENT SOURCE OF: vitamin A, vitamin C, vitamin K

GOOD SOURCE OF: fiber, calcium, potassium, vitamin E, riboflavin, folate, phosphorus, zinc, selenium, copper, manganese

supercharger

Oranges supercharge this recipe even more by providing fiber, potassium, vitamin C, and folate.

This salad is a showstopper. Not only are the colors of the tomatoes, beets, and oranges (if you supercharge it) stunning, the flavors with the creamy ricotta cheese are a match made in heaven. Add a sprinkle of fresh herbs and a drizzle of olive oil and this dish is truly memorable. This salad is bursting with nutrients to boost your energy, enhance your mood, and sharpen your focus. But the best part of all: it takes only 12 minutes to make!

¾ cup part-skim ricotta cheese

2 heirloom tomatoes, sliced

2 packaged (store-bought) cooked beets (about 5.5 ounces total), sliced

3 tablespoons extra-virgin olive oil

2 tablespoons white balsamic or white wine vinegar

½ cup packed roughly chopped fresh herbs, such as basil, mint, and flat-leaf parsley

¾ teaspoon flaked sea salt

½ teaspoon freshly ground black pepper

⅓ cup pine nuts, toasted (optional)

supercharger

1 large or 2 small oranges, cut into sections or round slices (optional)

Smear the ricotta cheese in a few dollops across a large rimmed serving platter. Pat the tomatoes and beets dry of excess liquid with paper towels. Arrange the tomatoes, beets, and oranges (if using) around and on top of the ricotta. Drizzle with the olive oil and balsamic vinegar, sprinkle with the herbs, salt, pepper, and toasted pine nuts (if using). Serve immediately.

PER SERVING: Calories 200; Total Fat 14 g (Sat Fat 3.5 g); Protein 7 g; Carb 13 g; Fiber 3 g; Cholesterol 15 mg; Sodium 520 mg; Total Sugar 8 g (Added Sugar 0 g)

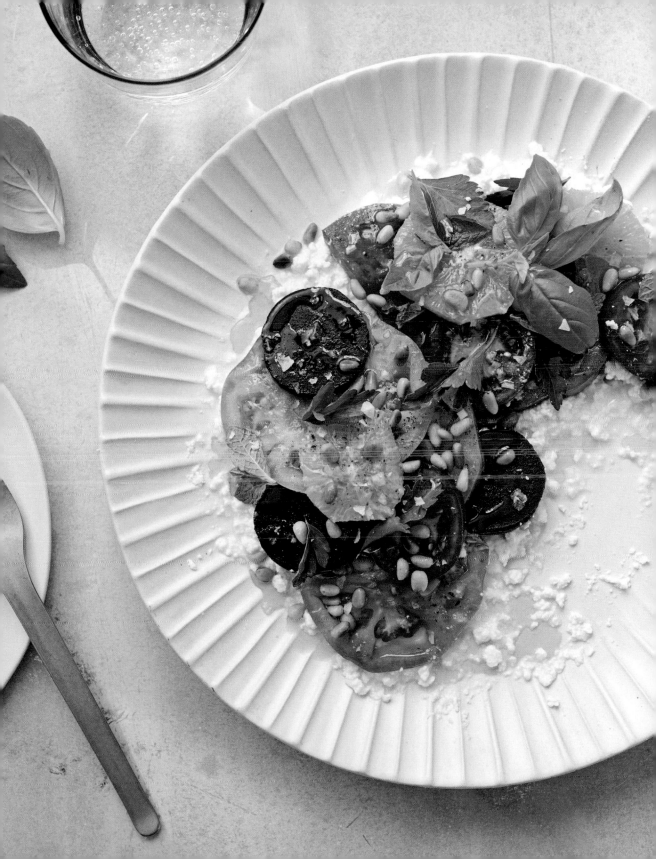

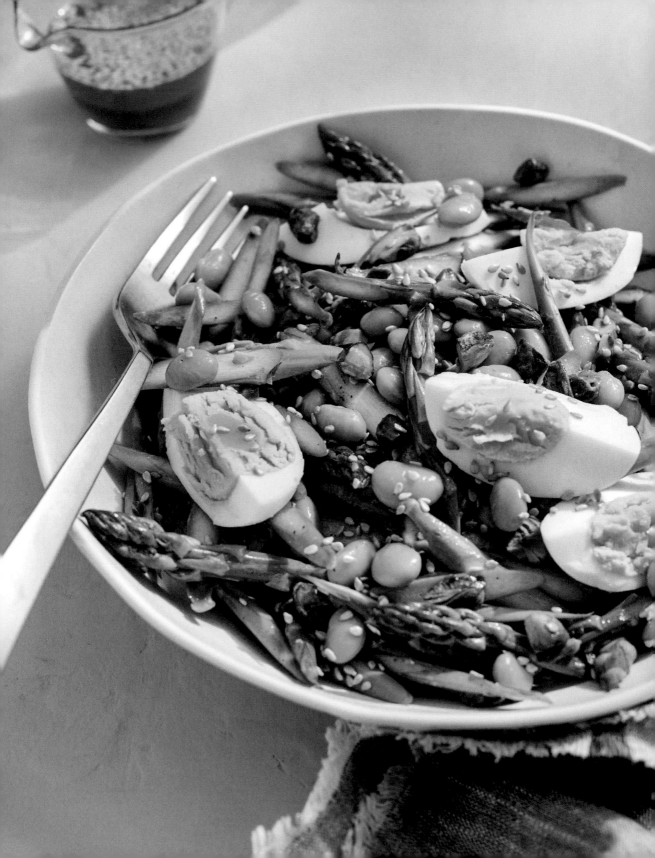

raw asparagus
& edamame salad
with sesame lime dressing

This Asian-inspired salad is a spring delight, and packed with foods to boost your mood and energy. Asparagus provides feel-good nutrients, like tryptophan, folate, B vitamins, and fiber. Its green counterparts, edamame and pistachios, add plant-based protein and crunch. Supercharge this salad with a hard-boiled egg or your favorite protein, or embellish with other additions like grated carrots, hearts of palm, avocado, or even shaved red cabbage.

● Vegetarian
● Gluten-Free (if using tamari)
● Dairy-Free
● Great for Leftovers (dressing only)
● 30 Minutes or Less

sesame lime dressing

⅓ cup avocado oil or sunflower oil

Juice of 2 limes (about ¼ cup)

2 tablespoons rice vinegar

1 tablespoon plus 1 teaspoon toasted sesame oil

1 tablespoon plus 1 teaspoon reduced-sodium soy sauce or tamari

1 tablespoon plus 1 teaspoon honey

¼ teaspoon sea salt

1 tablespoon white sesame seeds, raw or toasted (optional)

salad

2 cups frozen shelled edamame

1 pound thin asparagus spears

⅓ cup shelled salted roasted pistachios, roughly chopped

¾ teaspoon sea salt

½ teaspoon freshly ground black pepper

1 tablespoon mixed black and white sesame seeds, raw or toasted (optional)

supercharger

4 hard-boiled eggs, chopped (optional)

TIME SAVER: Use bottled organic or natural sesame or sesame ginger dressing.

TIP: Steaming eggs to make hard-boiled eggs is easier than boiling them. If supercharging this recipe, you can learn how to steam eggs on page 206

TIP: For best results, cut the asparagus spears on the bias (on a diagonal) so that the slices are about 2 inches long and ¼ inch wide at their fattest part. However, if you prefer not to cut them, blanch the asparagus stalks for 30 seconds and shock in an ice-water bath. Or do a quick sauté.

SERVINGS: 4

SERVING SIZE: 1½ cups

PREP TIME: 22 minutes (including dressing prep; not including hard-boiled egg prep)

COOK TIME: 5 minutes

EXCELLENT SOURCE OF: fiber, iron, vitamin A, vitamin C, vitamin K, copper

GOOD SOURCE OF: calcium, potassium, thiamin, riboflavin, folate

Make the dressing: Whisk all of the ingredients for the dressing in a small bowl or shake in a jar and set aside. Note: You'll have more dressing than needed for this salad. (Makes about 1 cup.)

Make the salad: Prepare an ice water bath by filling a large bowl with cold water and ice. Prepare the edamame according to package directions. Drain and place the edamame in the ice water bath to cool.

While holding the woody stem end, cut the asparagus on a very sharp angle (on the bias) into extra-thin slices and place in a large mixing bowl. Compost (or discard) the woody ends. Drain the edamame well

(recipe continues)

supercharger
Hard-boiled eggs supercharge this recipe even more by providing protein, choline, riboflavin, vitamin B_{12}, phosphorus, and selenium.

and pat dry. Add the edamame to the bowl with the asparagus. Add about ½ cup of the dressing, or to taste, and the pistachios and toss until everything is very well coated. (Reserve the remaining dressing for another use.) Add the hard-boiled eggs (if using), salt, and pepper and gently toss until just combined.

Transfer the salad to a serving dish or to plates, sprinkle with the sesame seeds, if desired, and serve.

The salad is best day of, but keeps well in the fridge, covered, for up to 1 day. If making in advance, wait until serving time to add the pistachios and sesame seeds. Dressing will last in an airtight container, such as a mason jar, in the refrigerator for up to 1 week.

PER SERVING (with ½ cup dressing, total): Calories 300; Total Fat 20 g (Sat Fat 2.5 g); Protein 17 g; Carb 20 g; Fiber 8 g; Cholesterol 0 mg; Sodium 640 mg; Total Sugar 7 g (Added Sugar 3 g)

roasted coriander cauliflower & tomatoes

This side dish is so full of flavor, it's bound to wow you! You'll enjoy the contrasting textures of the chewy bite of the roasted cauliflower, the juiciness of the tomatoes, and the crunchiness of the almonds. The larger the grape tomatoes, the better. Using "natural" almonds means you're also getting the nutrient-rich almond skin, and adding a dash of black pepper helps increase the absorption of the turmeric, which offers anti-inflammatory benefits. For a meal rather than a side dish, top your favorite cooked ancient grains with these roasted veggies for a yummy grain bowl. Or for a protein packed bowl, serve over a lentil- or bean-based "rice."

¼ cup unsalted, unsweetened cashew butter

Grated zest and juice of 1 small lemon (about 2 tablespoons juice)

1 large garlic clove, grated (on a microplane or box grater)

2 tablespoons unrefined (virgin) coconut oil, melted

2 teaspoons ground coriander

¼ teaspoon ground turmeric

¾ teaspoon sea salt

½ teaspoon freshly ground black pepper

1 medium head cauliflower, cut into 1½- to 2-inch florets (about 6 cups florets)

1 cup large grape tomatoes

¼ cup roughly chopped fresh cilantro leaves with tender stems

supercharger

¼ cup sliced natural almonds (optional)

● Vegan
● Gluten-Free
● Dairy-Free
● No Added Sugar

TIME SAVERS: Purchase cauliflower florets instead of the whole head of cauliflower. Use almond butter as a swap if you can't find cashew butter.

TIP: If using sliced almonds, pan-toast them for extra nuttiness. Place in a dry skillet over medium heat, turning frequently, until golden and fragrant, 3 to 5 minutes.

TIP: Buy a 16-ounce package of grape tomatoes and pick out the largest. Then toss the remaining smaller tomatoes into a salad or use in a salsa.

SERVINGS: 4

SERVING SIZE: 1 rounded cup

PREP TIME: 15 minutes

COOK TIME: 30 minutes

EXCELLENT SOURCE OF: vitamin C, vitamin K, vitamin B₆, folate, pantothenic acid, copper, manganese

GOOD SOURCE OF: fiber, iron, potassium, vitamin A, thiamin, riboflavin, phosphorus, magnesium, zinc

Preheat the oven to 450°F. Line a large rimmed baking sheet with parchment paper.

In a large bowl, whisk together the cashew butter, lemon zest, lemon juice, garlic, coconut oil, and 1½ teaspoons water until a thick sauce forms. Add the coriander, turmeric, salt, and pepper and whisk until well

(recipe continues)

supercharger

Almonds
supercharge this
recipe even more by
providing protein, fiber,
healthy fats, vitamin E,
and antioxidants.

incorporated. Add the cauliflower florets and whole tomatoes and stir with a flexible spatula or spoonula until the vegetables are fully and evenly coated with the sauce.

Evenly arrange the coated cauliflower and tomatoes in a single layer on the lined baking sheet. (Vegetable pieces should not touch each other, to allow for proper roasting.) Roast until the cauliflower is lightly browned, about 20 minutes. Remove from the oven, turn just the cauliflower over using tongs, and then continue roasting until the cauliflower is richly browned, about 10 minutes more.

To serve, top with the sliced almonds (if using), and cilantro. This dish is best enjoyed right away, but any leftovers can be stored in an airtight container in the fridge for up to 2 days.

PER SERVING: Calories 200; Total Fat 15 g (Sat Fat 7 g); Protein 6 g; Carb 15 g; Fiber 4 g; Cholesterol 0 mg; Sodium 480 mg; Total Sugar 5 g (Added Sugar 0 g)

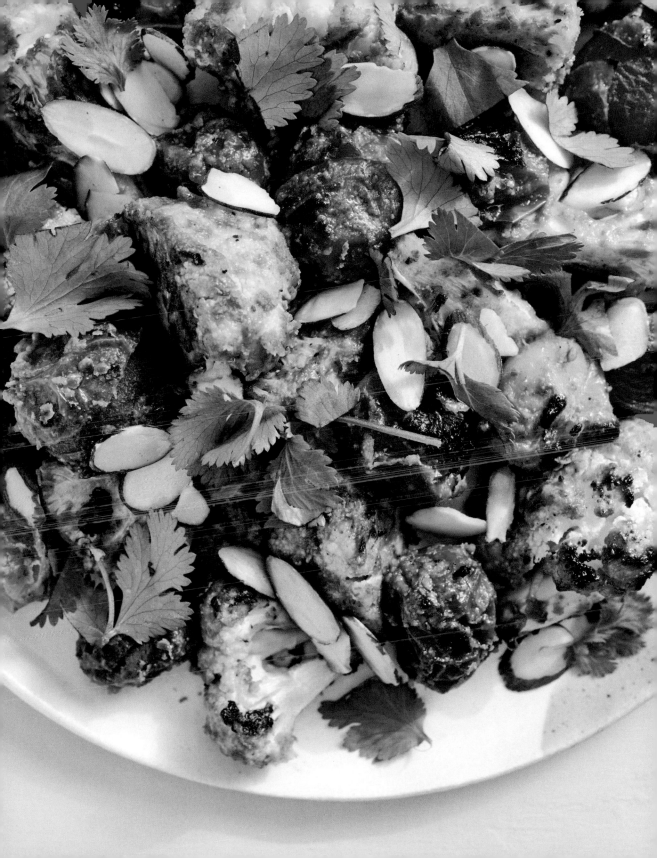

gruyère, grains & roasted zucchini squash bake

● Vegetarian
● Nut-Free
● No Added Sugar
● Great for Leftovers

TIME SAVER: Use a quick-cooking option, like 10-minute farro or 90-second brown rice.

TIP: Don't have panko? Use crushed crackers. Or toast whole-grain bread and chop it in a food processor.

SERVINGS: 8

SERVING SIZE: 1 cup

PREP TIME: 18 minutes (with precooked grains)

COOK TIME: 45 minutes

EXCELLENT SOURCE OF: calcium, vitamin A, riboflavin, vitamin B$_{12}$, phosphorus

GOOD SOURCE OF: vitamin C, pantothenic acid, zinc, selenium

PER SERVING: Calories 270; Total Fat 14 g (Sat Fat 6 g); Protein 14 g; Carb 24 g; Fiber 2 g; Cholesterol 35 mg; Sodium 600 mg; Total Sugar 4 g (Added Sugar 0 g)

supercharger

Mushrooms supercharge this recipe even more by providing B vitamins, selenium, and copper.

This side dish is one of my favorites for a gathering of family or friends. It's actually one of those rare cozy, casserole-style bakes that's light enough for spring or summer entertaining—but you can make it any time of the year. It's kind of like a baked risotto—or in this case, a farrotto!

4 cups cooked farro or other whole grains, chilled

1¼ teaspoons sea salt, divided

½ cup minced fresh chives (about 1 ounce)

2 medium (8-ounce) zucchini, cut into ⅓-inch-thick coins

2 tablespoons extra-virgin olive oil

2½ teaspoons organic cornstarch

1¾ cups 1% fat milk or plain unsweetened almond milk, divided

1 tablespoon minced fresh thyme leaves

2 large garlic cloves, minced

8 ounces Gruyère cheese, shredded (2 cups)

⅓ cup panko bread crumbs

Grated zest of 1 large lemon (optional)

supercharger

1 cup finely chopped baby bella mushrooms (optional)

Preheat the oven to 425°F.

In a 10-inch round or other 2-quart-capacity baking dish, stir the grains and mushrooms (if using), with ½ teaspoon of the salt, then arrange in an even layer. Evenly top with the chives and then zucchini coins, overlapping the zucchini if needed. Sprinkle with the olive oil and ¼ teaspoon of the salt. Press down with a spatula to pack ingredients.

In a medium saucepan off heat, whisk together the cornstarch and ½ cup of the milk until smooth. Place over medium-high heat and whisk in the remaining 1¼ cups milk, the thyme, garlic, and remaining ½ teaspoon salt. Cook, whisking occasionally, until the mixture is frothy and just beginning to boil, about 5 minutes. (Do not bring to a full boil.) Remove from heat. Stir in the Gruyère until just melted.

Evenly pour the Gruyère sauce over the zucchini and grains in the baking dish. Sprinkle with the panko. Bake until the topping is browned and crisp, about 40 minutes. Let stand for 5 minutes, sprinkle with lemon zest, if using, and serve.

The casserole keeps well in the fridge, covered, for up to 4 days. Gently reheat in the oven or microwave.

kale caesar salad

A healthful twist on a classic, this simple salad features a tangy, thick, and creamy dressing that's actually vegan. The capers act like anchovies in the salad, and the textures and taste of the greens are well balanced with a combination of kale and romaine. But my favorite part may be the panko topping. Panko bread crumbs, olive oil, and nutritional yeast add a nutty, cheesy, and slightly crunchy element that reminds me of homemade croutons.

vegan caesar dressing

¾ cup vegan mayonnaise

Juice of 1 lemon (about 3 tablespoons)

1 tablespoon white miso paste

1 tablespoon nutritional yeast

2 large garlic cloves, minced

¼ teaspoon sea salt

1 teaspoon freshly ground black pepper

panko topping

2 teaspoons extra-virgin olive oil

½ cup gluten-free panko bread crumbs

1 tablespoon nutritional yeast

salad

1 small (8-ounce) bunch green kale, very finely chopped with stems and thick ribs removed (6 cups packed)

1 small (8-ounce) head romaine lettuce, cored and shredded (6 cups packed)

3 tablespoons drained capers, chopped

supercharger

½ cup sliced natural almonds, toasted (optional)

- Vegan
- Gluten-Free
- Dairy-Free
- No Added Sugar (look for vegan mayo without added sugar)
- 30 Minutes or Less

TIME SAVERS: Purchase bags of chopped kale and chopped romaine.

TIP: Transform this salad into an entree by adding grilled salmon, scallops, or shrimp—or, keep it vegan with roasted chickpeas.

TIP: If supercharging this salad with sliced almonds, pan-toast them for extra nuttiness. Place in a dry skillet over medium heat, turning frequently, until golden and fragrant, 3 to 5 minutes.

SERVINGS: 6

SERVING SIZE: 2 cups

PREP TIME: 18 minutes (including dressing prep)

COOK TIME: 2½ minutes

EXCELLENT SOURCE OF: fiber, vitamin A, vitamin C, vitamin K, thiamin, riboflavin, niacin, vitamin B_6, folate, vitamin B_{12}, pantothenic acid, copper

GOOD SOURCE OF: manganese

Make the dressing: Shake all of the ingredients for the dressing in a jar or other sealable container until the miso paste is fully incorporated. Set aside. (Makes 1 cup.)

Make the topping: Preheat a small skillet over medium-high heat. Add the olive oil and bread crumbs and toast while stirring until the bread crumbs turn golden brown, about 2½ minutes. Transfer the bread crumbs to a bowl, stir in the nutritional yeast, and set aside.

Make the salad: In a large mixing bowl or rimmed serving platter, combine the kale, romaine, capers, and dressing and toss to fully and generously coat the salad.

Transfer the salad to plates or serve on the platter. Sprinkle with the panko topping and almonds (if using), and serve immediately.

Wait until serving time to sprinkle with the panko topping and almonds.

PER SERVING (WITH DRESSING): Calories 260; Total Fat 22 g (Sat Fat 3.5 g); Protein 12 g; Carb 19 g; Fiber 11 g; Cholesterol 0 mg; Sodium 480 mg; Total Sugar 3 g (Added Sugar 0 g)

supercharger

Almonds
supercharge this recipe even more by providing protein, fiber, healthy fats, vitamin E, and antioxidants.

snacks
&
sweets

"cheesy" lemon pepper popcorn

This perky recipe is like glammed-up cheese popcorn . . . no cheese required. Contrary to popular belief, popcorn is not "junk" food. Popcorn is made from a flint corn, which is a whole grain. One trick to keeping it wholesome is to pop it in a heart-healthful oil, like you'll do here with extra-virgin olive oil. The other trick is to be mindful of your flavorings. Here they're nutritional yeast flakes, lemon zest, garlic powder, sea salt, and lots of freshly ground black pepper.

⅓ cup nutritional yeast flakes

1½ teaspoons grated lemon zest

½ teaspoon garlic powder

½ teaspoon sea salt

1 teaspoon freshly ground black pepper

¼ cup extra-virgin olive oil, divided

½ cup unpopped popcorn kernels

supercharger

1 cup salted roasted chickpeas (optional)

Combine the nutritional yeast flakes and lemon zest in a large mixing bowl. Using the back of a large spoon or a flexible spatula, smash the lemon zest into the nutritional yeast flakes to infuse a strong lemony flavor into the flakes while breaking them up into a powdery consistency. Add the garlic powder, salt, and pepper and stir to combine. Set aside.

Heat 3 tablespoons of the olive oil in a large saucepan with a lid over medium-high heat. To test the heat, drop 3 popcorn kernels into the pan. Once these kernels pop, add the rest of the kernels to the pan in a single layer, making sure all kernels are fully coated with the oil. Cover with the lid and cook for 1 minute undisturbed, and then begin shaking the pan every 15 to 20 seconds once the kernels are popping frequently to prevent the popcorn from burning. Once the popping slows to about 1 pop every 3 seconds, transfer the popped kernels to the mixing bowl with the seasoning mixture. Drizzle with the remaining 1 tablespoon of olive oil. Stir or toss the popcorn well to make sure it is evenly coated with the seasoning mixture. Add the roasted chickpeas, if using, and stir or toss until evenly combined. Taste to adjust for seasoning. Serve warm and enjoy!

Popcorn keeps well in an airtight container for up 3 days.

PER SERVING: Calories 190; Total Fat 12 g (Sat Fat 1.5 g); Protein 5 g; Carb 17 g; Fiber 4 g; Cholesterol 0 mg; Sodium 230 mg; Total Sugar 0 g (Added Sugar 0 g)

- Vegan
- Gluten-Free
- Nut-Free
- Dairy-Free
- No Added Sugar
- Kid-Friendly
- Great for Leftovers
- 15 Minutes or Less

TIP: Periodically change up the supercharger by tossing this flavorful popcorn with roasted edamame or pistachios.

SERVINGS: 5

SERVING SIZE: 2 cups

PREP TIME: 8 minutes

COOK TIME: 5 minutes

EXCELLENT SOURCE OF: thiamin, riboflavin, niacin, vitamin B_6, folate, vitamin B_{12}, pantothenic acid

GOOD SOURCE OF: fiber, zinc, selenium, manganese

supercharger

Roasted chickpeas supercharge this recipe even more by providing protein, fiber, healthy fats, iron, folate, and phosphorus.

put-it-on-everything dip or spread

- Vegan
- Gluten-Free
- Dairy-Free
- Great for Leftovers
- 15 Minutes or Less

TIP: Since you'll have leftover canned white beans, store them in a sealed container in the fridge for later use in the Smashed White Bean and Radish Toast on page 141.

TIP: For bonus plant-based nutrition and intrigue, use iced unsweetened green tea instead of water in the recipe.

SERVINGS: 10

SERVING SIZE: ¼ cup

PREP TIME: 15 minutes

COOK TIME: 0 minutes

EXCELLENT SOURCE OF: vitamin E, thiamin, riboflavin, niacin, vitamin B_6, vitamin B_{12}, copper, manganese

GOOD SOURCE OF: fiber, folate, pantothenic acid, magnesium

This simple dip or spread recipe offers lots of flavor depth with an earthy spice accent from chili powder, cumin, and coriander. Using the spinach supercharger gives it a lovely natural green tone, and the fresh lemon zest provides a bright note. Unlike store-bought dips and spreads that are loaded with unhealthy ingredients, this recipe provides protein and fiber for staying power, along with an array of nutrients to help you feel and function at your best. This is a great recipe for everyday use—as well as a party dip. It tastes extra awesome after the flavors marry, so you can make it the day before a party. Chilling the dip thickens it up slightly, too.

1 cup whole raw almonds

⅔ cup water

⅔ cup drained canned low-sodium white beans (such as cannellini, navy, or great northern beans)

Grated zest and juice of 2 large lemons (about 6 tablespoons juice)

¼ cup avocado oil or sunflower oil

2 tablespoons nutritional yeast

2 large garlic cloves, peeled

2 tablespoons reduced-sodium soy sauce or Bragg liquid aminos or coconut aminos

½ teaspoon chili powder

¼ teaspoon ground cumin

¼ teaspoon ground coriander

½ teaspoon sea salt, or to taste

supercharger

1½ cups packed fresh baby spinach (optional)

Place all ingredients except the lemon zest in a high-powered blender, including the spinach, if using. Blend on low speed for 1 minute. Scrape down the sides of the blender. Then blend on high speed until creamy, about 3 minutes more. Taste and blend in your desired amount of the lemon zest.

Using a flexible spatula, transfer the spread to a sealable container and chill until ready to serve. Serve in a bowl alongside your favorite crudité platter, crackers, or fresh baguette. Spread will last in an airtight container in the fridge for up to 3 days.

PER SERVING: Calories 160; Total Fat 13 g (Sat Fat 1 g); Protein 5 g; Carb 9 g; Fiber 3 g; Cholesterol 0 mg; Sodium 290 mg; Total Sugar 1 g (Added Sugar 0 g)

supercharger

Spinach supercharges this recipe even more by providing vitamin A, vitamin C, vitamin K, folate, and manganese.

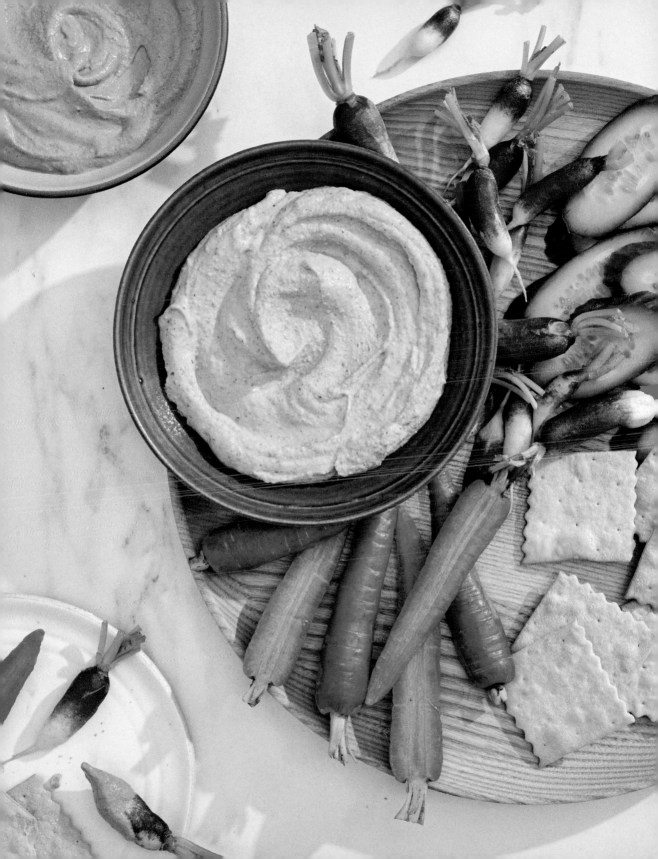

hummus deviled eggs

Deviled eggs have been served in American households for an entire century! That certainly makes them a classic. And while the traditional version will always be loved, this recipe offers a thoroughly modern twist. For the filling, mayo is out; creamy hummus is in. If you want to make the recipe party ready, use a piping bag to fill the egg whites, but serving them homestyle is just as tasty. And don't forget the finishing touch—you'll be sprinkling the deviled eggs with pickled vegetables to add an inviting splash of color along with probiotics, which are beneficial for gut health.

- Vegetarian
- Gluten-Free
- Nut-Free
- Dairy-Free
- No Added Sugar
- Kid-Friendly
- Great for Leftovers
- 30 Minutes or Less

TIME SAVERS: Use store-bought hard-boiled eggs. You can skip the entire first step and save about 15 minutes. When a recipe calls for lemon juice but not the zest, like this one, you can use bottled organic 100% lemon juice.

SERVINGS: 6

SERVING SIZE: 2 deviled egg halves

PREP TIME: 12 minutes

COOK TIME: 15 minutes

EXCELLENT SOURCE OF: riboflavin, vitamin B_{12}, selenium

GOOD SOURCE OF: vitamin A, folate, pantothenic acid, phosphorus, zinc, copper

supercharger

Pickled vegetables supercharge this recipe even more by providing fiber, B vitamins, and probiotics, along with a fun pop of color.

6 large eggs

½ cup store-bought hummus or Fresh Herb Hummus on page 131

2 teaspoons Dijon mustard

1 teaspoon lemon juice

¼ teaspoon sea salt

½ teaspoon freshly ground black pepper

⅛ teaspoon paprika

2 tablespoons minced fresh chives

supercharger

¼ cup chopped pickled veggies of choice, such as beets, carrots, or purple cabbage (optional)

Add 1 inch of water to a medium saucepan and set up a steamer basket. Bring the water to a boil over high heat (making sure the water isn't touching the basket) and carefully add the eggs to the steamer basket. Cover and steam on high for 10 to 12 minutes. (Note: The pan will be extra hot.) Carefully rinse the eggs in cold water and peel under cold running water. (If you don't have a steamer basket, go ahead and hard-boil these eggs using your preferred method.)

Slice the hard-boiled eggs in half lengthwise. Remove the yolks and place them in a small mixing bowl. Fully mash the yolks with a fork. Add the hummus and stir until the mixture is creamy. Add the mustard, lemon juice, salt, and pepper and stir until smooth and creamy.

Using a small spoon or piping bag, fill the center of each egg white half with the hummus mixture. Sprinkle with the paprika, pickled veggies (if using), and chives, and serve chilled.

The deviled eggs keep well in an airtight container in the fridge for up to 4 days.

PER SERVING: Calories 110; Total Fat 7 g (Sat Fat 2 g); Protein 8 g; Carb 3 g; Fiber 1 g; Cholesterol 185 mg; Sodium 290 mg; Total Sugar >1 g (Added Sugar 0 g)

five-ingredient chocolate chip banana oat bites

These easy-to-make bites are the perfect marriage of banana muffins and chocolate chip cookies. If you add blueberries, it's like a hint of blueberry pie, too! These cookies are sweet enough to enjoy as dessert, yet healthful enough to savor at breakfast time. You'll find plant-based protein and plenty of fiber here, along with mood-boosting ingredients and an aroma to match. I love making a batch of these and stashing half in the freezer.

● Vegan
● Gluten-Free (use certified gluten-free oats)
● Dairy-Free
● Kid-Friendly
● Great for Leftovers

SERVINGS: 16 (yields 16 cookies, or 20 cookies with blueberries)

SERVING SIZE: 1 cookie

PREP TIME: 12 minutes

COOK TIME: 30 minutes

EXCELLENT SOURCE OF: vitamin E, riboflavin, copper, manganese

GOOD SOURCE OF: fiber, magnesium

1¾ cups mashed extra-ripe banana (from about 3 large bananas)

1 cup creamy unsalted, unsweetened almond butter

¼ cup plus 2 tablespoons maple syrup

¾ teaspoon sea salt

2½ cups old-fashioned rolled oats

¼ cup mini dark chocolate chips or finely chopped bittersweet chocolate

supercharger

1 cup fresh blueberries (optional)

Preheat the oven to 350°F. Line two large baking sheets with parchment paper.

Stir together the mashed banana, almond butter, maple syrup, and salt in a large bowl until well combined. Add the oats, chocolate chips, and blueberries (if using), and stir until evenly combined. Using a muffin scooper, ice cream scooper, or ¼-cup measure, scoop the batter into mounds on the lined baking sheets to make a total of 16 cookie mounds (or 20 mounds if using blueberries). Bake until the cookies are lightly firm to the touch and browned on the bottoms, 28 to 30 minutes, rotating the baking sheets halfway through. Let cookies cool on the baking sheets on racks for at least 5 minutes before serving. Cookies will firm up slightly as they cool.

Store cooled cookies in an airtight container in the fridge for up to 3 days, or in the freezer for up to 1 month.

PER SERVING: Calories 200; Total Fat 11 g (Sat Fat 1.5 g); Protein 5 g; Carb 24 g; Fiber 4 g; Cholesterol 0 mg; Sodium 110 mg; Total Sugar 10 g (Added Sugar 6 g)

supercharger

Blueberries supercharge this recipe even more by providing fiber, potassium, vitamin C, vitamin K, and manganese.

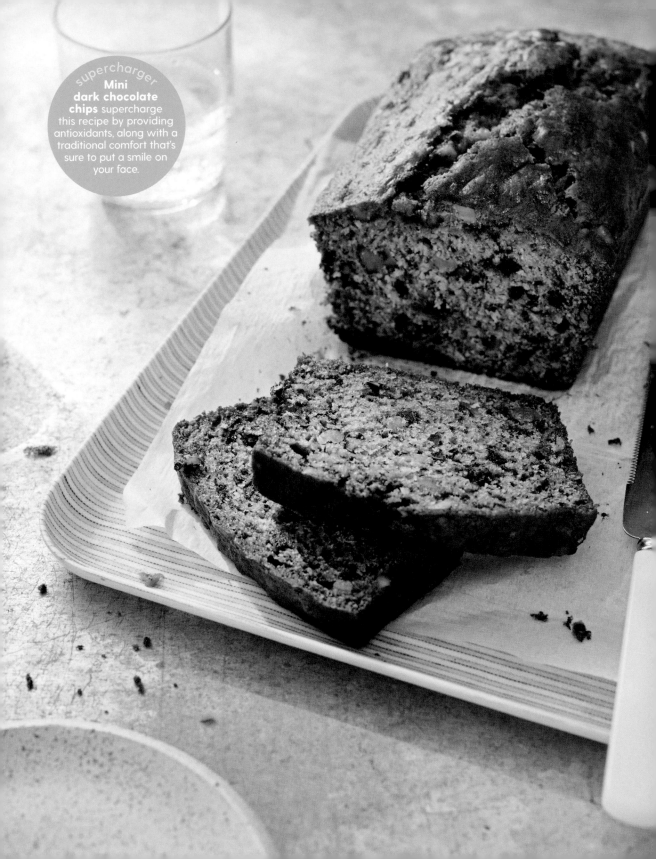

supercharger

Mini dark chocolate chips supercharge this recipe by providing antioxidants, along with a traditional comfort that's sure to put a smile on your face.

better-than-ever banana bread

This recipe is the perfect use for those brown-spotted bananas, which offer mood- and energy-boosting nutrients. Even if you don't need banana bread today, freeze it for when you do. It freezes sooo well. Supercharge it with mini dark chocolate chips (at least 60% cacao) for a classic comfort food fix, along with some additional antioxidants. For breakfast, be sure to pair it with some protein, such as yogurt or a latte.

2⅓ cups mashed extra-ripe banana (from about 5 medium bananas)

¾ cup plus 2 tablespoons organic granulated cane sugar, divided

½ cup avocado oil or sunflower oil

2 teaspoons pure vanilla extract

2 large eggs

2 cups unbleached all-purpose flour

1 teaspoon baking powder

1 teaspoon baking soda

1 teaspoon sea salt

1 cup walnut halves, chopped

supercharger

⅓ cup mini dark chocolate chips (optional)

Preheat the oven to 350°F. Spritz a 9 x 5-inch loaf pan with cooking oil spray and line with parchment paper. (The cooking oil spray will help the parchment paper stick to the pan nicely.)

In a large bowl, combine the mashed bananas, ¾ cup of the sugar, the oil, and the vanilla and whisk until the oil is incorporated. Add the eggs and whisk to combine.

Using a sifter or mesh strainer, sift the flour, baking powder, baking soda, and salt into the bowl with the wet ingredients. Stir until all of the dry ingredients are absorbed, being careful not to overmix.

Fold in the chopped walnuts and chocolate chips (if using), then pour the batter into the lined loaf pan. Sprinkle the batter with the remaining 2 tablespoons of sugar and bake until the center is firm and no longer gooey, seventy to eighty minutes. (Hint: Insert a paring knife or toothpick in the center; when the bread is done, it will come out clean.) Let cool for at least 20 minutes in the pan on a rack before slicing.

Banana bread will keep well in a sealed container for up to 1 day at room temperature, in the fridge for up to 1 week, or in the freezer for up to 3 months.

● Vegetarian (or vegan if using flax egg replacer)
● Dairy-Free
● Kid-Friendly
● Great for Leftovers

TIP: After enjoying the fresh-baked slices right away, chill in the fridge or slice and freeze; then thaw or warm up in the microwave as you wish . . . or even enjoy semifrozen slices like a dessert!

TIP: For bonus fiber, swap in 2 cups whole wheat pastry flour for the 2 cups of unbleached all-purpose flour.

TO MAKE VEGAN: Instead of 2 eggs, stir together 2 tablespoons ground flaxseed and 5 tablespoons of water in a small bowl. Let stand for at least 10 minutes before adding to the recipe.

SERVINGS: 12

SERVING SIZE: 1 slice

PREP TIME: 15 minutes

COOK TIME: Seventy to eighty minutes (plus 20 minutes standing time)

EXCELLENT SOURCE OF: thiamin, selenium, copper, manganese

GOOD SOURCE OF: riboflavin, niacin, vitamin B$_6$, folate

PER SERVING: Calories 320; Total Fat 16 g (Sat Fat 2 g); Protein 5 g; Carb 42 g; Fiber 2 g; Cholesterol 25 mg; Sodium 310 mg; Total Sugar 20 g (Added Sugar 14 g)

mini lemon blueberry muffins

● Vegetarian
● Kid-Friendly
● Great for Leftovers

TIP: If you can't find whole wheat pastry flour, try a mixture of flours, such as 1⅓ cups all-purpose flour plus ⅓ cup whole wheat flour.

TIP: If you choose to bake with frozen blueberries, you don't need to thaw them!

SERVINGS: 12 (yields 24 mini muffins)

SERVING SIZE: 2 mini muffins

PREP TIME: 20 minutes

COOK TIME: 15 minutes

GOOD SOURCE OF: fiber

PER SERVING: Calories 180; Total Fat 7 g (Sat Fat 1 g); Protein 4 g; Carb 25 g; Fiber 3 g; Cholesterol 30 mg; Sodium 115 mg; Total Sugar 11 g (Added Sugar 9 g)

These right-size muffins have a lovely balance of lemon, almond, and blueberry flavors. While muffins are sometimes cupcakes in disguise, these actually offer wholesome nutrition. Instead of bleached white flour, they're made with a whole wheat pastry flour, so they count as a source of whole grains while still being light in texture. And instead of butter, you'll use a combination of yogurt and avocado oil to cut down on saturated fat.

1⅔ cups whole wheat pastry flour

1 tablespoon baking powder

½ teaspoon sea salt

½ cup plus 1 tablespoon organic granulated cane sugar, divided

1 tablespoon grated lemon zest

⅓ cup avocado oil or sunflower oil

Juice of 1 small lemon (about 2 tablespoons)

½ cup plain 2% fat Greek yogurt or plant-based Greek-style yogurt

2 large eggs, lightly beaten

1 teaspoon pure vanilla extract

½ teaspoon pure almond extract

1 cup fresh or frozen blueberries

supercharger

2 tablespoons white chia seeds (optional)

Preheat the oven to 350°F and line a 24-cup mini muffin pan with mini muffin liners.

Whisk the flour, baking powder, salt, and chia seeds (if using) in a medium mixing bowl to combine. Set aside.

Combine ½ cup of the sugar and the lemon zest in a large mixing bowl. Using a flexible silicone spatula or the back of a large spoon, smash the lemon zest with the sugar to infuse. Add the oil and stir to combine. Then add the lemon juice, Greek yogurt, eggs, and extracts and stir until creamy. Add the dry ingredients and stir until evenly incorporated and smooth. Gently fold in the blueberries. Spoon the batter into the prepared muffin tins, completely filling the cups, about 2 tablespoons of batter in each. Sprinkle the tops with the remaining 1 tablespoon sugar.

Bake until the muffins are domed and spring back lightly to the touch, 15 to 18 minutes. (Note: Do not look for brownness.) Let muffins cool in the pan on a rack.

Store muffins covered at room temperature for up to 2 days or in the fridge for up to 5 days, or in the freezer for up to 3 months.

supercharger

Chia seeds supercharge this recipe even more by providing protein, fiber, healthy fats, calcium, phosphorus, and magnesium.

peanut butter stuffed dates

These are my go-to snack when I'm hungry midday and need something healthy in a hurry. Plus, they satisfy my desire for something sweet. The bigger, juicier, and plumper the dates, the better. When the dates are served cold, they are slightly firmer and the chewy texture is a delicious contrast to the super-smooth peanut butter. You can swap out the peanut butter for almond butter, cashew butter, or tahini. If using the dark chocolate supercharger, choose one that's at least 60% cacao.

12 large Medjool dates

¼ cup creamy natural peanut butter

½ teaspoon flaked sea salt

supercharger

1 ounce dark chocolate, chopped (optional)

Line a small baking tray or cutting board with parchment for easy cleanup.

Using your fingers, gently tear each date in half lengthwise, but don't pull them completely apart. If your dates are not already pitted, remove the pits to create a small cavity.

Spoon about 1 teaspoon of the peanut butter into the center of each date. Top each peanut butter center with a big pinch of the chopped dark chocolate (if using), and a little pinch of the sea salt. Gently close the dates back up and place onto the lined tray.

Enjoy right away or refrigerate for at least 30 minutes and serve chilled. You can stash in the freezer for later, too. To freeze, place in a freezer bag or airtight freezer container for up to 2 months.

PER SERVING: Calories 200; Total Fat 6 g (Sat Fat 1 g); Protein 3 g; Carb 38 g; Fiber 4 g; Cholesterol 0 mg; Sodium 200 mg; Total Sugar 33 g (Added Sugar 0 g)

- Vegan
- Gluten-Free
- Dairy-Free
- No Added Sugar
- Kid-Friendly
- 15 Minutes or Less

TIP: Additional topping favorites include freeze-dried raspberries, chopped pistachios, pomegranate arils, shredded coconut, or a dusting of cocoa or cinnamon.

TIP: If you're a fan of frozen candy bars, freeze these stuffed dates and indulge in them when they're semifrozen. Remove from the freezer and let stand for a few minutes before taking a bite.

SERVINGS: 6

SERVING SIZE: 2 stuffed dates

PREP TIME: 10 minutes

COOK TIME: 0 minutes

EXCELLENT SOURCE OF: copper

GOOD SOURCE OF: fiber, niacin, vitamin B$_6$, pantothenic acid, magnesium, manganese

supercharger

Dark chocolate supercharges this recipe even more by providing antioxidants, along with a traditional comfort that's sure to put a smile on your face.

pumpkin spice almond butter balls

- ● Vegan (without honey)
- ● Gluten-Free (choose certified gluten-free oats)
- ● Dairy-Free
- ● Kid-Friendly
- ● Great for Leftovers
- ● 30 Minutes or Less

TIP: You won't need an entire can of pumpkin puree for this recipe. Save the leftovers for smoothies, oatmeal, and pumpkin spice lattes. You can also freeze it in an ice cube tray for later use.

SERVINGS: 14

SERVING SIZE: 2 balls

PREP TIME: 20 minutes

COOK TIME: 0 minutes

EXCELLENT SOURCE OF: vitamin A

GOOD SOURCE OF: fiber, vitamin E, riboflavin, copper, manganese

This sweet treat will remind you of a luxurious pumpkin pie, albeit in a healthier way! One of the main ingredients is just as you'd expect: pumpkin puree. That makes these goodies like sneaky little veggie bombs. They've also got whole-grain oats and almond butter for texture and nutrition, and no refined sugar. To make them, you simply whirl everything together in a food processor, roll into balls, and stash in the fridge. Then they're ready to pop into your mouth as a snack anytime you need a quick pick-me-up.

1⅓ cups old-fashioned rolled oats

½ cup creamy unsalted, unsweetened almond butter

½ cup pumpkin puree

8 large Medjool dates, pitted

2 tablespoons maple syrup or honey

1¼ teaspoons pumpkin pie spice or cinnamon

½ teaspoon pure vanilla extract

¾ teaspoon sea salt

supercharger

⅓ cup shelled hemp seeds (optional)

In the bowl of a food processor, process the oats on high speed until a flour is formed, about 1 minute. Add the remaining ingredients and process on high speed until a cohesive and sticky dough forms, at least 1½ minutes, scraping the sides of the food processor bowl as needed. Taste to adjust for overall sweetness and seasoning.

Line a tray or baking sheet with parchment paper. One at a time, roll the mixture by hand into 28 balls, about 1 tablespoon each, then roll in the hemp seeds, if using, to coat. (Hint: For easier rolling, slightly moisten your hands with a damp paper towel.) Place the balls onto the prepared tray and place it in the fridge for at least 30 minutes, to firm up the balls. Enjoy at room temperature or chilled, straight from the fridge.

The balls keep well in an airtight container in the fridge for up to 1 week.

PER SERVING: Calories 140; Total Fat 6 g (Sat Fat 0 g); Protein 3 g; Carb 21 g; Fiber 3 g; Cholesterol 0 mg; Sodium 125 mg; Total Sugar 13 g (Added Sugar 2 g)

supercharger

Hemp seeds supercharge this recipe even more by providing protein, fiber, healthy fats, iron, vitamin E, and magnesium.

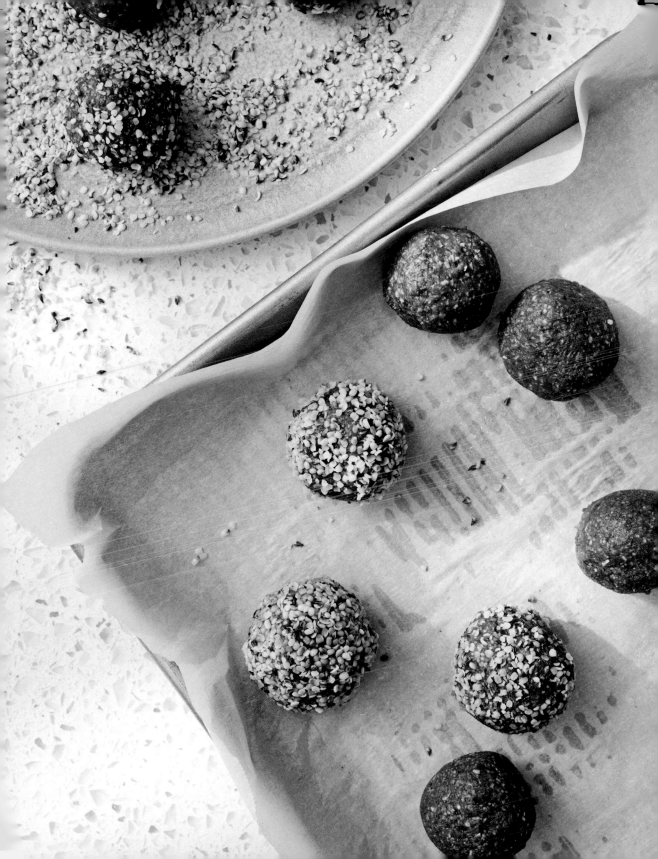

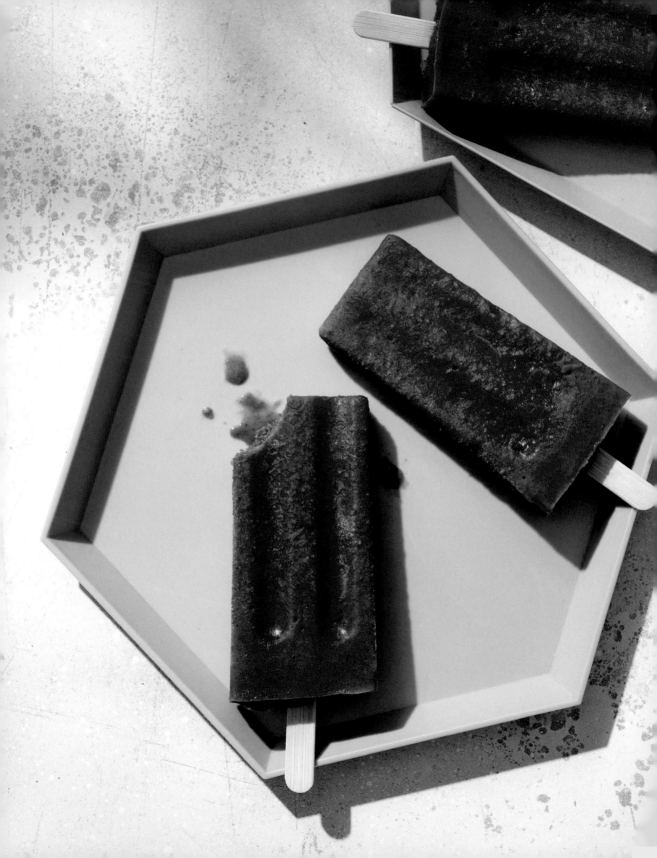

mango beet
ice pops

These ice pops are the prettiest fuchsia ever, due mainly to the betalain (red pigment) in beets, which also has potential anti-inflammatory properties. Greek yogurt adds a creamy texture and mood-boosting nutrients, while mango may help with digestion, immunity, and eyesight. Supercharge these treats with chia seeds for added protein and fiber. Since they freeze well, make a batch to keep on hand.

● Vegetarian
● Gluten-Free
● Nut-Free
● Kid-Friendly
● 15 Minutes or Less

TIP: Be sure your mangoes are fully ripened for optimal natural sweetness. In fact, if they are super sweet you can do without the honey or coconut nectar.

SERVINGS: 6

SERVING SIZE: 1 (4-ounce) popsicle

PREP TIME: 10 minutes (plus at least 4 hours of freezing time)

COOK TIME: 0 minutes

EXCELLENT SOURCE OF: vitamin A, vitamin C

GOOD SOURCE OF: folate, copper

2¼ cups chopped ripe fresh mango (from about 2 medium mangoes)

¾ cup chopped (store-bought) cooked beets (about 4.5 ounces)

½ cup plain 2% fat Greek yogurt

Juice of 1 lime (about 2 tablespoons)

2 tablespoons honey or coconut nectar

supercharger

1 tablespoon chia seeds (optional)

Combine the mango, beets, yogurt, lime juice, and honey in a high-powered blender and blend on high until bright pink, creamy, and smooth, about 2 minutes. If using, add the chia seeds and pulse just until incorporated throughout. Pour into 6 ice pop molds, about 4 ounces each.

Insert popsicle sticks and freeze until solid, at least 4 hours.

Ice pops keep well frozen for up to 1 month.

PER SERVING: Calories 90; Total Fat 0.5 g (Sat Fat 0 g); Protein 3 g; Carb 21 g; Fiber 2 g; Cholesterol 0 mg; Sodium 25 mg; Total Sugar 19 g (Added Sugar 6 g)

supercharger

Chia seeds supercharge this recipe even more by providing protein, fiber, healthy fats, calcium, phosphorus, and magnesium.

green tea soft serve

- Vegan
- Gluten-Free
- Nut-Free
- Dairy-Free
- No Added Sugar
- Kid-Friendly
- Great for Leftovers
- 15 Minutes or Less (plus freezer time)

TIME SAVER: Freeze a batch of ripe bananas each month so they're ready anytime you'd like to make this recipe or blend up a quick smoothie.

TIP: The soft serve can be frozen and then reprocessed for the same texture.

SERVINGS: 2

SERVING SIZE: 1 cup

PREP TIME: 5 minutes (plus banana freezing time)

COOK TIME: 0 minutes

EXCELLENT SOURCE OF: fiber, potassium, vitamin A, vitamin C, vitamin B$_6$, copper, manganese

GOOD SOURCE OF: riboflavin, folate, pantothenic acid, magnesium

This two-ingredient "nice" cream couldn't be easier to make, and it's one of my favorites to have on hand when I'm in need of a cool and energizing treat. A refreshing and mild matcha flavor is blended with plenty of banana goodness. If you love matcha, add more matcha powder to please your taste buds. This doesn't melt like traditional soft serve ice cream, so don't worry about working extra speedily from food processor to serving. Add almond butter or shelled hemp seeds for an extra punch of healthy fats and protein, or enjoy as is!

3 large ripe bananas, peeled, sliced into 1-inch pieces, and frozen

1 tablespoon culinary matcha green tea powder

supercharger
2 tablespoons cacao nibs (optional)

Remove the sliced frozen bananas from the freezer and let stand for 3 minutes to slightly thaw. Place the bananas and matcha powder in the bowl of a food processor and process until the texture resembles creamy soft serve ice cream, scraping down the sides of the bowl as needed. Pulse or stir in the cacao nibs, if using.

Serve immediately or place in the freezer to firm up slightly for 10 minutes. The soft serve keeps well in the freezer for up to 1 month.

PER SERVING: Calories 210; Total Fat 1 g (Sat Fat 0 g); Protein 4 g; Carb 50 g; Fiber 8 g; Cholesterol 0 mg; Sodium 0 mg; Total Sugar 25 g (Added Sugar 0 g)

supercharger

Cacao nibs supercharge this recipe even more by providing fiber, magnesium, and antioxidants.

fudgy avocado walnut brownies

When people ask me about my favorite indulgence, I have only one answer: chocolate! The richer, the better, which is why these avocado brownies fit the bill. Made with some better-for-you ingredients—like whole wheat pastry flour, sunflower oil, walnuts, and avocado—they add a bit more nutrition than your average brownie. Supercharge them with banana slices for an added touch of mood-boosting nutrients and comfort. This is a "big batch" recipe; so it's ideal for when you need to bake a goody for a party, too!

- Vegetarian
- Dairy-Free (choose dairy-free chocolate chips)
- Kid-Friendly
- Great for Leftovers

TIP: Whole wheat pastry flour is a whole-grain soft white wheat flour—which is perfect for baking. If you can't find it, simply use all-purpose flour. Or for gluten-free, flourless brownies, use coconut flour instead of whole wheat pastry flour.

SERVINGS: 24

SERVING SIZE: 1 brownie

PREP TIME: 18 minutes

COOK TIME: 30 minutes

EXCELLENT SOURCE OF: zinc, copper

GOOD SOURCE OF: fiber, iron, vitamin K, manganese

⅔ cup whole wheat pastry flour

½ cup unsweetened cocoa powder

½ teaspoon sea salt

1 ripe large avocado, sliced

7 large eggs

½ teaspoon pure vanilla extract

1¼ cups organic granulated cane sugar

14 ounces bittersweet chocolate chips (about 60% cacao)

¾ cup sunflower oil

1 cup walnut halves and pieces, chopped

supercharger

3 small bananas, sliced (optional)

Heat the oven to 350°F. Line the bottom of a 9 x 13-inch baking pan with parchment paper. In a small bowl, whisk or sift together the flour, cocoa powder, and salt until well combined. Set aside.

In a large mixer bowl, blend the avocado with an electric mixer on medium speed until whipped and velvety smooth. Add the eggs, vanilla, and sugar and mix just until well combined and smooth. Set aside.

Gently melt the chocolate with the oil in a double boiler (or medium mixing bowl placed over hot water) until smooth.

Stir the melted chocolate mixture into the whipped avocado-egg mixture until fully combined. Sprinkle in the cocoa mixture and stir everything together until well combined. Fold in the walnuts. Pour and spread the batter into the prepared pan. Bake until springy to the touch about 2 inches from the sides, about 30 minutes.

Cool completely in the pan on a rack. Cut into 24 brownies, top with banana slices (if using), and serve. Store covered in the fridge for up to 5 days or freeze individual, well-wrapped brownies for up to 3 months.

PER SERVING: Calories 240; Total Fat 17 g (Sat Fat 5 g); Protein 4 g; Carb 21 g; Fiber 3 g; Cholesterol 45 mg; Sodium 60 mg; Total Sugar 14 g (Added Sugar 14 g)

supercharger

Bananas supercharge this recipe even more by providing fiber, potassium, vitamin C, and vitamin B$_6$.

sleepy almond chamomile cookies

- Vegetarian
- Gluten-Free (choose certified gluten-free oats)
- Dairy-Free
- Kid-Friendly

TIP: If you don't have loose-leaf chamomile tea, simply use the tea leaves emptied from 3 chamomile tea bags.

TIP: Cookies will actually appear *underbaked* when you remove them from the oven, but will firm up afterward.

TO MAKE VEGAN: Substitute 3 tablespoons water and 1 tablespoon chia seeds or ground flaxseed for 1 egg; substitute vegan butter or coconut oil for butter.

SERVINGS: 16 (yields 16 cookies)

SERVING SIZE: 1 cookie

PREP TIME: 20 minutes

COOK TIME: 14 minutes

GOOD SOURCE OF: fiber, vitamin E

These soft bedtime cookies even smell soothing. The key is to avoid overbaking them. Almonds are a natural source of magnesium, an essential mineral that helps the body relax. And these cookies celebrate almonds in three ways—with almond flour, sliced almonds, and almond extract. Chamomile is an herb that contains the flavonoid apigenin, which is thought to help calm the body and induce sleep. And oats are rich in melatonin, a hormone that helps regulate circadian rhythm. But most important, these cookies are much tastier than a sleeping pill.

2½ cups old-fashioned rolled oats

1½ cups almond flour

2 tablespoons dry loose-leaf chamomile tea

½ teaspoon sea salt

½ cup honey

6 tablespoons unsalted butter, softened, or vegan butter alternative

1 large egg

¾ teaspoon pure almond extract

⅓ cup plus 2 tablespoons sliced natural almonds, divided

supercharger

⅓ cup dried cranberries, chopped (optional)

Preheat the oven to 350°F and line a large baking sheet with parchment paper.

Process the oats in a food processor and on high speed until a finely ground oat flour forms. Add the almond flour, chamomile tea, and salt and pulse to incorporate. Add the honey, butter, egg, and almond extract and process on low speed until the mixture just forms a dough. Transfer to a bowl and fold in ⅓ cup of the almonds and the cranberries (if using).

Scoop then roll the dough by hand into 16 balls, about 2 rounded tablespoons each. (Hint: Wipe hands clean throughout with a damp paper towel.) Arrange the balls on the prepared baking sheet, spaced about 1 inch apart. Press the remaining sliced almonds on top, about 3 or 4 pieces per ball.

Bake for 10 to 11 minutes; cookies will appear undercooked but will firm up when they cool. (The cookies are meant to be soft; if you overbake them, they will become dry and biscotti-like.) Let cookies cool on the baking sheet on a rack for at least 20 minutes. They're best enjoyed at room temperature the day they are made, or store them in an airtight container in the fridge for up to 1 week.

PER SERVING: Calories 200; Total Fat 12 g (Sat Fat 3.5 g); Protein 5 g; Carb 20 g; Fiber 3 g; Cholesterol 25 mg; Sodium 80 mg; Total Sugar 10 g (Added Sugar 8 g)

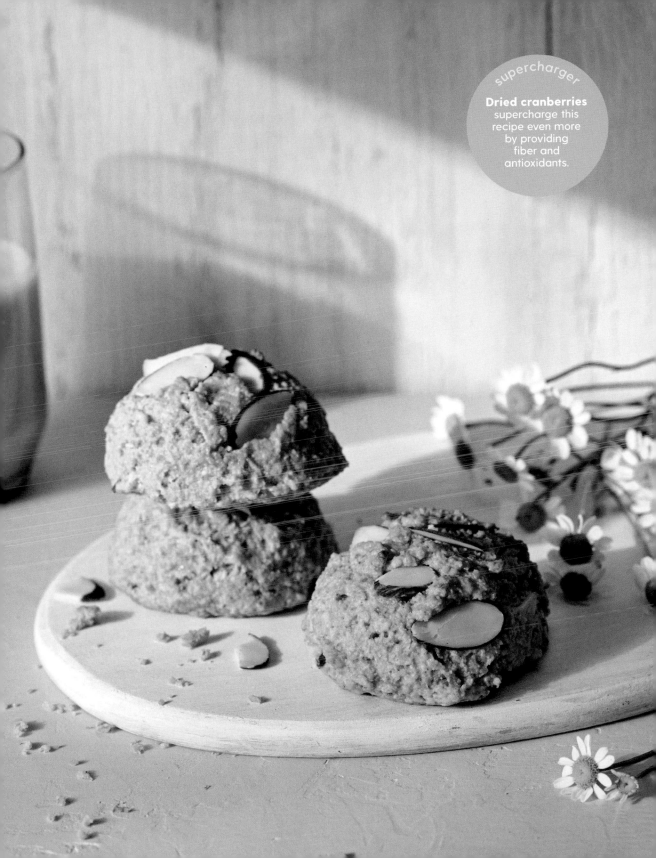

supercharger

Dried cranberries
supercharge this
recipe even more
by providing
fiber and
antioxidants.

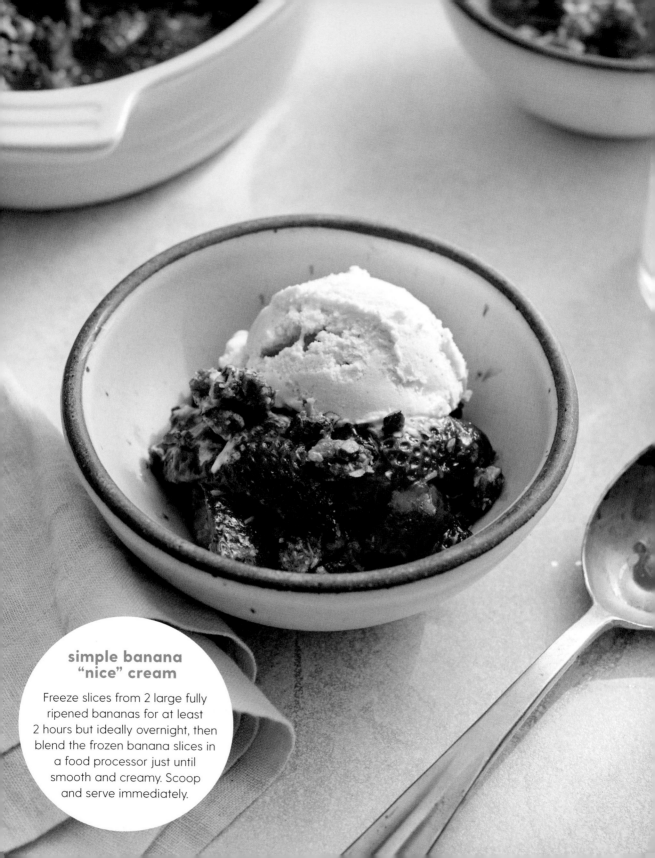

simple banana "nice" cream

Freeze slices from 2 large fully ripened bananas for at least 2 hours but ideally overnight, then blend the frozen banana slices in a food processor just until smooth and creamy. Scoop and serve immediately.

strawberry pecan crisp

This is a must-make recipe when strawberries are in season. Simply tossing fresh strawberries with the pecan topping tastes almost like pecan pie, without all the added sugar and calories you'd find in a traditional pastry! Strawberries provide energizing nutrients like vitamin C and fiber, while pecans offer protein and healthy fats. Supercharge it with coconut flakes for additional texture, flavor, and nutrition. Top the crisp with your favorite ice cream, or a whip up some simple banana "nice" cream for a healthier twist. Kid-friendly and classically comforting, this is a staple dessert recipe the whole family will enjoy.

● Vegetarian
● Gluten-Free
(choose certified gluten-free oat flour)
● Kid-Friendly

TIP: If you like, you can bake individual strawberry crisps in 8-ounce ramekins so everyone has their own dessert.

SERVINGS: 4

SERVING SIZE: ¾ cup

PREP TIME: 15 minutes

COOK TIME: 25 minutes

EXCELLENT SOURCE OF: vitamin C, copper, manganese

GOOD SOURCE OF: fiber, thiamin, magnesium, zinc

strawberry filling

14 ounces fresh strawberries, stemmed and quartered (about 2½ cups quartered)

2 teaspoons honey or coconut nectar

½ teaspoon pure vanilla extract

1¼ teaspoons organic cornstarch

pecan topping

¾ cup chopped pecans

2 tablespoons oat or coconut flour

¼ teaspoon ground cinnamon

⅛ teaspoon sea salt

1 tablespoon honey or coconut nectar

2 teaspoons unsalted butter, chilled, cut into 12 tiny cubes

Vanilla bean ice cream or banana "nice" cream, for serving (optional)

supercharger

3 tablespoons unsweetened dried coconut flakes (optional)

Preheat the oven to 375°F. Spritz a 1- or 1¼-quart baking dish with cooking spray.

Make the filling: In a medium bowl, stir together the strawberries, honey, and vanilla to combine. Sprinkle with the cornstarch and stir to fully coat. Transfer to the baking dish and pat into an even layer.

Make the topping: In a small bowl, stir together the pecans, flour, cinnamon, salt, and coconut flakes (if using) until combined. Drizzle with the honey and stir until the mixture resembles a sticky granola cereal. Sprinkle the topping evenly over the strawberry mixture. Sprinkle with the butter.

Bake until the topping is browned and strawberries are fully softened, about 25 minutes. Scoop into small dessert dishes to serve while warm. If desired, top each with a scoop of ice cream or banana "nice" cream.

PER SERVING: Calories 240; Total Fat 17 g (Sat Fat 2.5 g); Protein 3 g; Carb 21 g; Fiber 4 g; Cholesterol 5 mg; Sodium 110 mg; Total Sugar 13 g (Added Sugar 7 g)

supercharger

Coconut flakes supercharge this recipe even more by providing fiber, selenium, and manganese.

acknowledgments

Every book represents the work of not only its author but also dozens of others who play pivotal roles behind the scenes. I'm grateful to so many people who helped make this book a reality:

First, thank you to my editors, Donna Loffredo and Danielle Curtis, who believed in this book from the beginning and had the vision and brilliance to make it even stronger.

Thank you to my literary agent, Linda Konner, for representing me and for finding such a lovely home for this book. Thanks also to the fantastically talented and dedicated Jennifer Chong and her team for the beautiful photography and for bringing the recipes to life.

Thanks also to my trusted and epically talented colleagues and friends for lending their expertise all along the way (and helping me prevent burnout in the process!): Stepfanie Romine, Sarah Powers, Jackie Newgent, Jori Finkel, Jodi Pfarr, and Ali McGowan.

A special thank-you to all the women who shared their real-life experiences and strategies with burnout; your stories enriched these pages.

And finally, to my family: Roman, Nicki, and Sienna. To my parents and greatest fans, Joanne and Bill. To Glenn, Maia, and Casner. To "Tante Lolie" for creating a loving blended family. To my in-laws, Ruth and Günter. Thank you all for a lifetime of love and support.

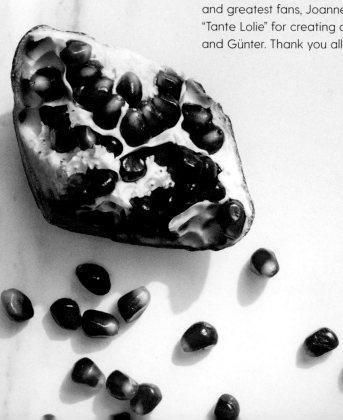

appendix 1

nutrition:
what to eat to beat burnout, and why

This section highlights how many essential nutrients influence the four core areas of burnout. While not an exhaustive list, it includes information on where to get these nutrients, what they do, and why they matter. The list starts with macronutrients (carbs, protein, fat), micronutrients, then moves on to essential vitamins, minerals, and more.

Complex carbs

TOP FOODS: whole grains, legumes and beans, nuts and seeds, fruits and vegetables

Mood: Feeds your brain and helps prevent "hangry feelings"; fiber helps digestion and your microbiome

Immunity: Fiber promotes an anti-inflammatory response in immune cells

Focus: Provides energy and fuel for the brain

Sleep: Supports better, deeper sleep

Complex carbohydrates pack in more nutrients than simple carbs and, due to their higher fiber content, take longer to break down. Complex carbs help stabilize blood sugar levels, which can also stabilize your mood. Fluctuations in blood glucose can cause your mood to change rapidly, leaving you irritable, low on energy, and feeling downright dreadful. The fiber in complex carbs also helps keep your gut healthy, which affects your mood, immune system, and more.

Lean protein

TOP FOODS: eggs, beans, peas, lentils, skinless white-meat poultry (chicken and turkey), fish and shellfish, pork loin, lean beef, bison, low-fat dairy (milk, yogurt, cottage cheese, cheese), soy milk, tofu, tempeh, soy beans (edamame), nuts and nut butters, seeds and seed butters

Mood: Helps with satiety and wards off "hanger"

Immunity: Necessary to repair and build tissues, including antibodies

Focus: Keeps your brain and nervous system healthy

Sleep: Amino acids make neurotransmitters that help sleep

Protein is necessary for healthy energy levels. It takes longer to digest than carbs, keeping your blood sugar steadier and providing lasting energy. Protein also affects hormones that control satiety, so when you eat enough of it, you can ward off "hanger" and stabilize blood sugar, which supports a better mood. Amino acids, the building blocks of protein, help repair and replenish tissue, and your body needs them to make certain neurotransmitters. Amino acids also play a role in maintaining a healthy mood, focus, and more.

Healthy fats

TOP FOODS: avocado, olives, oils (olive oil, avocado oil, sesame oil, and sunflower oil), fatty fish, whole eggs, tofu, nuts and seeds, dark chocolate

Mood: Help make hormones and support brain health

Immunity: Maintain a healthy immune system and absorb fat-soluble nutrients

Focus: Support brain function and memory

Sleep: Support healthy melatonin levels

Omega-3 fatty acids (DHA and EPA) are part of cell membranes, particularly in the brain, and eating foods like salmon and sardines has been shown to ease depression and boost mood. Low levels of DHA are linked to lower melatonin levels. Consuming fish rich in these fatty acids has also been found to help improve sleep.

Beyond omega-3s, the unsaturated fats found in plants like avocados, olives, and nuts may help keep inflammation at bay and reduce blood pressure, which are both important for brain health.

Eating enough healthy fat helps your immune system, too.

Folate

TOP FOODS: vegetables (especially dark green leafy ones like spinach, brussels sprouts, and asparagus), fruit and fruit juices, nuts, avocado, wheat germ, beans, peas, seafood, eggs, dairy products, meat, poultry, enriched grain products (such as cereals, flours, rice, pasta, bread)

Mood: Supports production of neurotransmitters

Immunity: Supports production of white blood cells and overall immune function

Folate plays a role in the production of dopamine and impacts other mood-related neurotransmitters, helping you keep calm and carry on. It also helps prevent neural tube defects in utero, supports cell growth and repair, and helps you regulate sleep patterns, especially as you age. A deficiency in folate levels has been tied to depression, too. Folate shortages are linked to a number of brain issues, including dementia and depression.

Folate is crucial for cell growth and DNA formation, and severe deficiencies are linked to increased cancer risks, among other diseases.

Vitamin B_6

TOP FOODS: fish, poultry, nuts, legumes, potatoes, fortified cereals, bananas, pistachios, avocado, spinach, flaxseeds, and sunflower seeds

Mood: Helps make neurotransmitters, including turning tryptophan into serotonin

Immunity: Supports immune function, including certain types of white blood cells

Sleep: Supports melatonin production

Vitamin B_6 helps the body make several neurotransmitters. Many of its roles also support protein metabolism. A B_6 deficiency will impact immune function by preventing proper growth, interfering with white blood cell production, and decreasing production of regulatory proteins.

Vitamin B_6 also helps your body manage your sleep-wake cycle and is needed to process, produce, and absorb melatonin.

Vitamin B_{12}

TOP FOODS: seafood (especially clams, mussels, crab, and sardines), liver, egg yolks, beef, cheese, and yogurt

Note: If you're vegan, you'll need to supplement this vitamin or consume fortified foods like nutritional yeast, soy milk, cereals, and breads.

Mood: Supports production of neurotransmitters

Immunity: Supports production of red blood cells and overall immune function

Focus: Healthy levels help support memory as we age

Sleep: A deficiency may impact the sleep-wake cycle

Vitamin B_{12} supports production of serotonin and dopamine, both of which help regulate mood. It is also required for red blood cell production and DNA formation. When you're low in vitamin B_{12}, it can lead to lower red blood cell production or impaired development of those vital cells. A deficiency is linked to memory loss, particularly in older adults, as well as brain atrophy. Vitamin B_{12} is believed to influence melatonin, and it may help improve your sleep-wake cycle so you awake feeling more refreshed.

Choline

TOP FOODS: egg yolks, liver, beef, chicken, pork, fish, milk, nuts, wheat germ, beans, peas, and cruciferous vegetables (broccoli, cauliflower, brussels sprouts, etc.)

Mood: Keeps energy, mood, and memory healthy and steady

Focus: Building block of acetylcholine (in charge of your working memory)

Choline is a B-vitamin-like nutrient that is essential. It helps produce neurotransmitters and improve mood. Only women's bodies are able to produce it—because choline synthesis is linked to estrogen. However, due to genetics, only half of us can convert estrogen into choline.

Choline helps make acetylcholine, a neurotransmitter necessary for memory and mood. That neurotransmitter plays a vital role in "working memory," which is your ability to remember information in the short term. Consuming choline has been studied as a way to prevent Alzheimer's, too.

Vitamin C

TOP FOODS: almost all fruits and vegetables, including oranges, lemons, strawberries, kiwi, bell peppers, tomatoes, and broccoli

Mood: Helps keep mood stable

Immunity: Supports immune cells and your epithelial barrier

Focus: Guards against inflammation that can lead to dementia

Sleep: Necessary for serotonin production

Vitamin C is a well-known antioxidant that assists the body's ability to make neurotransmitters, including dopamine, noradrenaline, and serotonin, which stabilize mood.

Your body needs vitamin C to maintain and repair all tissues, so it helps wounds and cuts heal. Plus, some of your infection-fighting white blood cells require vitamin C to function properly. Vitamin C also helps you manage stress. Your adrenal glands require it to make stress hormones, including cortisol. The more stressed you are, the more cortisol you produce—and the more vitamin C you need. But it has also been shown to improve tolerance to stress in lab settings. In addition, vitamin C may prevent the spikes in cortisol that happen when you're sleep-deprived.

Vitamin C functions as an antioxidant, protecting your brain from inflammation, which can raise your risk of developing cognitive issues, including Alzheimer's.

Vitamin A

TOP FOODS: sweet potatoes, spinach, carrots, melon, peppers, mangoes, eggs, fortified cereals and dairy, apricots, broccoli, yogurt, and salmon

Immunity: Necessary for cellular communication, protects the epithelial barrier and mucosal linings

Focus: Maintains mental flexibility and cognitive function as we age

Vitamin A strengthens your immune system to help fight off infections, and it plays a role in healthy development and growth. It protects your intestinal and other linings, and also helps regulate cell responses. The precursor to vitamin A, known most commonly as beta-carotene, is converted to vitamin A in the body.

Vitamin A serves as a signaling molecule in the brain as we grow. It plays a vital role in things like mental flexibility (neuroplasticity), the longevity of our neurons, and the resilience of our synapses, according to animal studies.

Vitamin D

TOP FOODS: fortified foods (like dairy products, orange juice, cereals, and milk alternatives), some fatty fish, beef liver, cheese, egg yolks

Note: Vitamin D is found in relatively few foods in two forms, D_2 and D_3. D_2 (ergocalciferol) is found in mushrooms and yeasts (as well as a few plants). D_3 (cholecalciferol) comes from animal foods. D_3 is more effective at raising levels of vitamin D in your blood, so if you choose D_2 sources, you'll need to consume more.

Mood: Helps make serotonin

Immunity: Modulates both innate and adaptive immune functions

Focus: Helps maintain cognitive function

Sleep: Low levels can put you at risk for sleep disorders

Vitamin D helps your body make serotonin—and it's sometimes called the "sunshine vitamin" because we can make it from sunlight. Most American adults have insufficient levels. When it comes to mood disorders, studies often show that people with depression who receive vitamin D supplements notice an improvement in their symptoms. Vitamin D deficiency can impair cognitive function, specifically the framework that forms and retains memories.

Vitamin D also regulates your immune system and supports your defenses against infections and diseases. It affects your innate immune system, especially in how your body responds to microbes. There's also some connection between deficiency and autoimmune diseases (including multiple sclerosis, rheumatoid arthritis, and inflammatory bowel disease).

Low vitamin D negatively affects several aspects of sleep, including quality, duration, and daytime sleepiness.

Vitamin E

TOP FOODS: sunflower seeds, almonds, hazelnuts, spinach, avocado, kiwi, mango, olive oil, sunflower oil, broccoli, peanuts, peanut butter, and wheat germ

Immunity: Functions as an antioxidant to protect immune cells, regulates processes like cell signaling and gene expression

Focus: Protects brain cells

Vitamin E acts as an antioxidant in the body, helping you ward off infection. It helps your cells live longer and may help mitigate damage from free radicals. It aids in cellular communication, and it supports the cells in the linings of your blood vessels, so they can stay free of buildup and let blood flow more freely.

In the brain, vitamin E exerts its antioxidant support to protect against Alzheimer's, dementia, stroke, and more.

Vitamin K

TOP FOODS: leafy greens, broccoli, brussels sprouts, asparagus, grapes, soybean oil, edamame, pine nuts, blueberries, pickles, sauerkraut, pomegranate juice

Immunity: Supports immune and inflammatory responses

Focus: Regulates calcium in the brain

Vitamin K plays key physiological roles in blood coagulation, bone metabolism, and the regulation of some enzyme systems. Plus, it can affect immune and inflammatory responses mediated by T cells. Studies have found links between vitamin K levels and inflammatory diseases and cancer, among other conditions

Studies have linked calcium to Alzheimer's, as the mineral can become imbalanced in brain cells of those suffering from the disease. That's where vitamin K comes in. Beyond its role in helping your blood clot, this fat-soluble nutrient regulates calcium and has anti-inflammatory effects.

● Calcium

TOP FOODS: sardines, dark leafy greens, soybeans (edamame), sesame seeds, enriched grains, fortified foods (such as dairy products, cereals, orange juice, and milk alternatives)

Mood: May ease PMS and support healthy mood

Focus: Supports memory and brain cells

Sleep: Helps boost melatonin

This essential mineral plays a crucial role in managing PMS (along with vitamin D). Estrogen, which is of course linked to PMS, is also connected to calcium production. Getting adequate amounts can help improve depression linked to PMS. Separately, low intake of calcium has been linked to depression.

Calcium plays a role in brain health, too. It aids cell signaling and helps regulate many functions of your neurons. Beyond that, it is also important for memory.

Deficiencies are linked to trouble falling asleep and less restful sleep—and it is yet another nutrient that helps boost melatonin. Calcium also helps maintain healthy blood pressure.

● Magnesium

TOP FOODS: nuts and seeds, cooked greens, bananas, avocado, dark chocolate, legumes, whole grains, some fatty fish (such as salmon, halibut, and mackerel)

Mood: May improve brain function to help ease anxiety and PMS

Focus: Boosts blood flow to brain

Sleep: Promotes relaxation, calms the nervous system, and maintains optimal GABA levels by binding to its receptors

Supplementing your diet with magnesium has been shown to help depression as well as fatigue and irritability. Plus, studies have found that magnesium (with vitamin B_6) can improve PMS symptoms.

Known for its role in relaxation, magnesium helps control the smooth muscle of your vascular system, which can boost blood flow (and thus oxygen) to your brain. Plus, exams of those who passed away with Alzheimer's showed lower levels of this essential mineral.

Research suggests a positive impact on sleep, too, since magnesium plays a role in maintaining GABA (a neurotransmitter that helps you relax and sleep soundly). Deficiencies are linked to restless leg syndrome, which can interfere with sleep.

Iron

TOP FOODS: beans, lentils, tofu, lean beef, turkey, chicken, oysters, baked potatoes, cashews, dark leafy greens, fortified cereals, whole and enriched grains

Note: Iron from animal sources (heme iron) is absorbed by the body more easily than the iron found in plant sources (non-heme iron). Pairing plant sources of iron with vitamin C can help increase absorption.

Mood: Supports energy levels and combats fatigue and depression

Immunity: Necessary for a healthy immune response and the production of red blood cells

Focus: Transports oxygen to the brain

Low iron can cause fatigue and depression—and deficiency is more common in women than in men, because we lose blood during our periods every month. Anemia (iron deficiency) causes symptoms similar to burnout: changes in mood, fatigue, loss of interest, and even depression. The proteins found in iron also help maintain healthy brain function and development. Anemia deprives your body—and brain—of adequate oxygen due to a shortage of healthy red blood cells.

Consuming too much or not enough iron can impact both your innate and your adaptive immune functions. When you have healthy levels of iron and use it effectively, harmful bacteria can't use the mineral for growth. And certain white blood cells fight off infection by carefully managing their iron levels.

Copper

TOP FOODS: oysters and lobster, spirulina, mushrooms, nuts and seeds, leafy greens, dark chocolate

Immunity: Helps maintain the immune system, necessary for red blood cell production

While your immune system needs copper, an essential mineral, for several processes, the research is still out on exactly why that is. We do know that copper deficiency can reduce levels of regulatory proteins and (most likely) T cell production.

Zinc

TOP FOODS: oysters, red meat, poultry, other types of shellfish, legumes (like lentils, chickpeas, and black beans), vegetables (including cruciferous ones and garlic)

Mood: Modulates the brain and body's response to stress

Immunity: Supports both the innate and adaptive immune systems, manages immune cell signals

Focus: Supports learning and memory

Sleep: A deficiency may impact the sleep-wake cycle

Zinc deficiency is linked to low energy, so making sure you get enough of this mineral can keep you feeling your best. Deficiency of this mineral can also cause symptoms including depression, ADHD, difficulties with learning and memory, seizures, aggression, and violence.

Zinc deficiencies can impair your immune system, and supplementing can stimulate some immune cells—and may shorten the duration of colds. Zinc also helps speed up wound healing and manages your immune system's inflammatory responses. It helps stimulate white blood cells that fight infections, including T cells and natural killer cells.

Beyond its importance within the immune system and wound healing, zinc also plays a crucial role in learning and memory. While the research is yet unclear as to exactly what zinc does, we do know that this essential mineral is tasked with regulating the release and supply of neurotransmitters, which is why it may help with sleep regulation as well.

Selenium

TOP FOODS: Brazil nuts, seafood, meat, poultry, eggs, dairy products, mushrooms, lentils, enriched grain foods

Mood: Helps maintain a healthy mood

Immunity: Functions as an antioxidant, protecting immune cells, and supports overall immune function

Optimal selenium levels yield optimal moods, according to one study of young adults. That study found that both too much and (especially) too little selenium were associated with depression. The antioxidant glutathione—sometimes called "the mother of all antioxidants" due to its very important roles in your body—needs selenium to function. Research has found a connection between low glutathione levels and mood disorders.

This essential mineral functions as an antioxidant, which reduces inflammation and protects your cells—including those in your immune system. Having ample levels of selenium can support your immune responses, while a deficiency can cause your immune system to slow down.

Probiotics and fermented foods

TOP FOODS: yogurt, kefir, sauerkraut, miso, kombucha, tempeh, kimchi, pickled vegetables, cheese

Mood: Nourishes your "gut brain" and supports mood

Immunity: Modulates the immune system within your gut

Focus: Aids cognitive function

Thanks to the probiotics they contain, fermented foods support the production of mood-regulating neurotransmitters (serotonin, dopamine, and GABA). Packed with healthy microbes, such as lactic acid bacteria, fermented foods have been shown to change brain activity and ease both stress and anxiety.

Speaking of your microbiome, the same probiotics that nurture your gut also boost your immune health. These good bugs fight the bad ones they encounter in your digestive tract, preventing them from entering your bloodstream or making you sick. Certain probiotics encourage production of antibodies, and they can also boost certain immune cells.

The gut-brain axis links the brain and the belly, and probiotics help keep both healthy. Since your gut is basically your second brain, probiotics support a healthy mood (as you read in chapter 3) and cognitive function, too. For example, people living with Alzheimer's saw improvements in their mental function after consuming probiotic-enriched milk for twelve weeks.

Prebiotics

TOP FOODS: fruits, vegetables, whole grains, nuts and nut butters, seeds and seed butters, chicory root, seaweed, cocoa, garlic

Mood: Reduces stress hormones and feeds the microbiome

Immunity: Nourishes the gut microbiome

Focus: Helps your gut bacteria support brain health as you age

Beyond soluble and insoluble fiber, described in chapter 2, foods like whole grains, nuts, seeds, fruits, and vegetables all contain prebiotic fibers. In addition to feeding your gut bacteria, some prebiotics can reduce stress hormones.

Prebiotics help modulate the immune system via the gut, and can shift the balance of the microbiome population. They directly affect the immune cells in the lining of your intestines, which can help your overall immune response as well as inflammation within the gut.

This fiber feeds the good bacteria in your gut, which may also support brain health as you age. And 2019 research revealed that maintaining a healthy, diverse gut microbiome during middle age can help your brain grow old gracefully—while preserving cognition and clarity.

Melatonin

TOP FOODS: tart cherries and tart cherry juice, asparagus, tomatoes, pomegranates, olives, grapes, broccoli, grains (oats, barley, rice), nuts, seeds

Sleep: Tells your body it's nighttime so you can relax and go to sleep

Tryptophan, as well as nutrients like calcium and vitamin B_6, help you produce melatonin, but you can also get this "sleep hormone" from certain foods. (See page 99 for more about tryptophan and sleep.) Melatonin doesn't have a soporific effect. Instead, it shifts you into a state that helps you ease your way toward sleep. Eating certain foods rich in melatonin before bed can help you take full advantage of the natural increase in this hormone that happens in the evening.

Caffeine

TOP FOODS: coffee, tea, dark chocolate

MOOD: Creates an alert, energized state

Focus: Provides mental clarity

While a moderate amount of caffeine (like a mug of morning java) can improve your mood, helping you feel more alert and energetic, too much can cause you to feel irritable, anxious, or jittery, and interrupt your sleep. If you're a tea lover, in addition to caffeine and antioxidants, tea provides L-theanine, an amino acid that can help you chill out without feeling groggy and boost your mood. Dark chocolate contains some caffeine (much less than coffee or tea), but it also contains flavonoids that boost blood flow (which may reduce fatigue) and your mood.

In moderate amounts, caffeine can serve as what's known as a nootropic, a substance that boosts brain function—including memory, focus, and concentration. That's why a cup of coffee can help you gain a little more mental clarity.

appendix 2

resources
where to find help when you need it

If you're feeling burned out, you are not alone! There's no shortage of resources that will provide you the information, strategies, and support you need to recharge your batteries. Here is a list of some of the best tools that will help you live the joyful life you deserve, even when those moments of stress, anxiety, and worry are simply unavoidable.

● Hotlines and On-Demand Help Services

Befrienders Worldwide: A global network of emotional support centers that offers an open space for any individual in distress to be heard. Support is available via phone or text message, in person, and online. https://www.befrienders.org

Crisis Text Line: A 24/7 text-accessible resource that connects individuals to real-life crisis counselors who are trained to bring texters from a hot moment to a calm state through active listening and collaborative problem solving. Counselors are trained in topics related to anxiety, emotional abuse, depression, suicide, school, and stress. Text HOME to 741741 (U.S.), 50808 (Canada) or 85258 (UK). https://www.crisistextline.org

Lifeline Chat: An on-demand, 24/7 service of the National Suicide Prevention Lifeline that connects individuals with counselors for emotional support and other services via web chat. Call 1-800-273-TALK (8255) for immediate support. https://suicidepreventionlifeline.org/chat

National Suicide Prevention Lifeline: A support site for suicidal individuals and their loved ones, survivors, mental health professionals, and others who care. If you are having thoughts of suicide, call the National Suicide Prevention Lifeline at 1-800-273-8255 (TALK). https://www.speakingofsuicide.com/resources

General Online Resources and E-courses

Anxiety and Depression Association of America—Managing Stress and Anxiety: An online database of resources like blog posts and webinars specific to different categories of anxiety, including anxiety in children and teens, severe weather, workplace anxiety, and sleep and anxiety. https://adaa.org/living-with-anxiety/managing-anxiety

Burnout Prevention and Treatment by HelpGuide—Techniques for Dealing with Overwhelming Stress: An online guide to mental health and wellness featuring signs/symptoms and lifestyle and dietary approaches to dealing with burnout. https://www.helpguide.org/articles/stress/burnout-prevention-and-recovery.htm

Center for Mindful Living—Free Mindfulness and Mindful Living Resources: A compilation of free audio and video resources, online programs, mindfulness teachings, and guided meditations that seek to build mindfulness and promote stress management. https://www.mindfullivingla.org/resources/mindfulness

InHerSight: A data-driven company that helps women find and improve organizations, advance diversity, and develop work-life balance. The InHerSight blog features contributor articles and resources to help women recognize and prevent burnout, manage stress, and make the most of their career objectives while juggling life's most stressful moments. https://inhersight.com/blog

Mind Tools: An online hub featuring blog posts, articles, infographics, videos, and other tools devoted to mental health and the workplace. Search "burnout," "stress," "anxiety," and other terms to find resources specific to your needs. https://www.mindtools.com

Thrive Global: An online platform dedicated to preventing burnout via blog posts, resources, and in-person events that are designed for individuals and organizations. Follow their social media for daily inspiration: @thrive on Instagram and Twitter and @thriveglb on Facebook. www.thriveglobal.com

Udemy: A compilation of 100,000 self-paced online video courses available for both desktop and smartphone, featuring videos on stress, anxiety, burnout in the workplace, and more. Courses start at $12.99 each. https://www.udemy.com

Unum Stress Awareness Module: A free short self-guided online workshop that walks managers through the physical and psychological effects of stress and the importance of stress management in the workplace. https://e-modules.unum.co.uk/stress-awareness

WellMD's Stress and Burnout Resource Hub: A compilation of resources designed for medical professionals, featuring screening tests and general information about different forms of stress—ranging from workplace and traumatic stress to burnout and resilience. https://wellmd.stanford.edu/test-yourself.html

● Mommy Burnout

Psyched Mommy: An online community that welcomes stories of honest motherhood experiences and provides free mental health resources that are specific to burnout in parents. Take advantage of a self-paced e-course with research-based recommendations about burnout for pregnant and postpartum women, or free mini courses, PDFs, and blog posts. Follow on Instagram and Facebook @psychedmommy. https://www .psychedmommy.com

Risen Motherhood: A faith-driven resource for Christian mothers that provides blog posts, downloadable resources, and podcasts specific to parenting with faith. Hear tips on how to manage roadblocks like postpartum depression, anxiety, and grief. Follow on Instagram and Facebook @risenmotherhood for daily inspiration. https://www.risen motherhood.com

● Resources for Black Women

Dive in Well: An organization offering digital classes on various wellness practices like breathwork and therapy sessions aimed at prioritizing self-care for Black women. https:// www.diveinwell.com

Melanin and Mental Health: An easy-to-navigate online directory that helps connect Black and Latinx women with mental health professionals in the area, while also raising awareness about the unique mental health challenges minorities face. Free resources include events for clinicians and community members as well as podcasts and blog posts. Follow on Instagram and Facebook at @melaninandmentalhealth. https:// www.melaninandmentalhealth.com

The Nap Ministry: An organization that examines the liberating power of naps. The group believes rest is a form of resistance and names sleep deprivation as a racial and social justice issue. Find immersive workshops and performance art that examines rest as a radical tool for community healing. https:// thenapministry.wordpress.com

Sista Afya Community Mental Wellness: A mental health organization that connects Black women to in-person and online mental health resources. Sista Afya achieves its mission through mental wellness education, including workshops, professional development opportunities, online resources, and event services. Follow on Instagram at @sistaafya for daily inspiration. https:// www.sistaafya.com

Therapy for Black Girls: A mental health hub devoted to changing the stigma around therapy by making mental health topics more relevant and accessible to Black women and girls. Resources include a therapy-match service, blog posts, podcast episodes, and merchandise devoted to encouraging the mental wellness of Black women. Follow on Instagram @therapyforblackgirls and subscribe to the *Therapy for Black Girls Podcast*. https:// therapyforblackgirls.com

Quizzes/Self-Assessments

Burnout Self-Test: A free online self-assessment developed by Mind Tools to determine if you have burnout or if you are at risk for developing stress-induced burnout. https://www.mindtools.com/pages/article/newTCS_08.htm

The Fried Quiz: A straightforward multiple-choice quiz that will help you decipher if your burnout is the source of your problems, followed by a set of suggested solutions that are tailored to your unique results. http://www.oprah.com/inspiration/burnout-quiz-assessment-test-fried-book_1

Apps

Calm: The #1 app for sleep, meditation, and relaxation. https://www.calm.com

Happify: Science-based activities and games to overcome worries and stress. https://happify.com

Headspace: Daily mindfulness and guided meditation activities. https://www.headspace.com

Time Out—Break Reminders: An app designed to interrupt long periods of screen time with friendly reminders to break. https://www.dejal.com

Tomato Timers: A free web-based site that provides intentional time management through the Pomodoro technique. http://www.tomatotimers.com

Videos and Podcasts

Talks for When You Feel Totally Burnt Out: A free database of TED Talks covering topics of stress, meditation, rest, recovery, and stillness. https://www.ted.com/playlists/245/talks_for_when_you_feel_totall

Happier with Gretchen Rubin: A podcast featuring relatable stories, implementable habits, and fun ideas to make your life a little happier. https://gretchenrubin.com/podcasts

The Happiness Lab **Podcast:** A deep dive into the science behind happiness with Dr. Laurie Santos. https://www.happinesslab.fm

Happiness Spells **Podcast:** A fun five-minute podcast that boosts happiness, gratitude, and creativity. https://www.happinessspells.com

The Struggle Bus **Podcast:** A biweekly advice show about mental health, self-care, and simply getting through the day. https://strugglebuspodcast.com

This Unmillennial Life **Podcast:** A personal journal podcast for women in midlife that covers topics you'd discuss with a friend. https://thisunmilleniallife.com

Unlocking Us with Brené Brown **Podcast:** An enlightening show that reflects the universal experiences of being human, from the bravest moments to the most brokenhearted. https://brenebrown.com/unlockingus/.

Chapter 1

13   **Meredith Corp and the Harris Poll** Meredith Corporation and Harris Poll, *Burnout Flashpoint*, 2019, http://online.fliphtml5.com/mseh/cfmp/#p=1.

13   **State of the American Workplace Report** Gallup, *State of the American Workplace Report*, 2017, https://www.gallup.com/workplace/238085/state-american-workplace-report-2017.aspx.

13   **"endorsement" of the World Health Organization** "Burn-Out an 'Occupational Phenomenon': International Classification of Diseases," World Health Organization, May 28, 2019, https://www.who.int/mental_health/evidence/burn-out/en/.

13   **first responders** J. A. Boscarino, C. R. Figley, and R. E. Adams, "Compassion Fatigue Following the September 11 Terrorist Attacks: A Study of Secondary Trauma among New York City Social Workers," *International Journal of Emergency Health* 6, no. 2 (2004): 57–66.

13   **social workers** Richard E. Adams, Joseph A. Boscarino, and Charles R. Figley, "Compassion Fatigue and Psychological Distress among Social Workers: A Validation Study," *American Journal of Orthopsychiatry* 76, no. 1 (2006): 103–8, https://doi.org/10.1037/0002-9432.76.1.103.

13   **clergy** Kevin J. Flannelly, Stephen B. Roberts, and Andrew J. Weaver, "Correlates of Compassion Fatigue and Burnout in Chaplains and Other Clergy Who Responded to the September 11th Attacks in New York City," *Journal of Pastoral Care & Counseling* 59, no. 3 (2005): 213–24, https://doi.org/10.1177/154230500505900304.

14   **increase in PTSD** Yuval Neria, Laura Digrande, and Ben G. Adams, "Posttraumatic Stress Disorder Following the September 11, 2001, Terrorist Attacks: A Review of the Literature among Highly Exposed Populations," *American Psychologist* 66, no. 6 (2011): 429–46, https://doi.org/10.1037/a0024791.

14   **piece by Arianna Huffington** Arianna Huffington, "We Are Never Going Back," Thrive Global, May 1, 2020, https://thriveglobal.com/stories/arianna-huffington-coronavirus-pandemic-opportunity-better-compassionate-world/?utm_source=Newsletter_AH.

14   **collapse back in 2007** Arianna Huffington, "10 Years Ago I Collapsed from Burnout and Exhaustion, and It's the Best Thing That Could Have Happened to Me," Thrive Global, April 6, 2017, https://medium.com/thrive-global/10-years-ago-i-collapsed-from-burnout-and-exhaustion-and-its-the-best-thing-that-could-have-b1409f16585d.

14   **specific subtypes for depression and anxiety** Leanne M. Williams, "Defining Biotypes for Depression and Anxiety based on Large-Scale Circuit Dysfunction: A Theoretical Review of the Evidence and Future Directions for Clinical Translation," *Depression and Anxiety* 34, no. 1 (2016): 9–24, https://doi.org/10.1002/da.22556.

14   **These "biotypes" are** https://neuroscience.stanford.edu/news/measuring-depression-wearables.

14   **our biotype—which can be observed** Leanne Williams, "How Understanding Your Biotype Can Help You Unlock Your Mental Health during a Pandemic," Thrive Global, May 1, 2020, https://thriveglobal.com/stories/coronavirus-stress-response-biotype-stanford-medicine-white-paper/?utm_source=Newsletter_General.

16   **Maslach Burnout Inventory** Christina Maslach, Susan Jackson, Michael Leiter, Wilmar Schaufeli, and Richard Schwab, "The Maslach Burnout Inventory-Test Manual," January 1996, https://www.researchgate.net/publication/256840539_The_Maslach_Burnout_Inventory-Test_Manual.

17   **a coping mechanism** "Feeling Grumpy 'Is Good for You,'" BBC News, November 5, 2009, http://news.bbc.co.uk/2/hi/health/8339647.stm.

17   **your brain shifts strategies** Joseph P. Forgas, "Affective Influences on Self-Disclosure: Mood Effects on the Intimacy and Reciprocity of Disclosing Personal Information," *Journal of Personality and Social Psychology* 100, no. 3 (2011): 449–61, https://doi.org/10.1037/a0021129.

17   **a study published in the** *European Journal of Preventive Cardiology* Parveen K. Garg, J'Neka S. Claxton, Elsayed Z. Soliman, Lin Y. Chen, Tené T. Lewis, Thomas Mosley, and Alvaro Alonso, "Associations of Anger, Vital Exhaustion, Anti-depressant Use, and Poor Social Ties with Incident Atrial Fibrillation: The Atherosclerosis Risk in Communities Study," *European Journal of Preventive Cardiology* 2020: 204748731989716, https://doi.org/10.1177/2047487319897163.

17   **coronary heart disease** "Coronary Heart Disease," National Heart, Lung, and Blood Institute, U.S. Department of Health and Human Services, accessed August 8, 2020, https://www.nhlbi.nih.gov/health-topics/coronary-heart-disease.

17   **a study by the American Friends of Tel Aviv University** Sharon Toker, Samuel Melamed, Shlomo Berliner, David Zeltser, and Itzhak Shapira, "Burnout and Risk of Coronary Heart Disease," *Psychosomatic Medicine* 74, no. 8 (2012): 840–47, https://doi.org/10.1097/psy.0b013e31826c3174.

18   **a study published in 2019** Heather M. Padilla, Mark Wilson, Robert J. Vandenberg, Marsha Davis, and Malissa A. Clark, "Health Behavior among Working Adults: Workload and Exhaustion Are Associated with Nutrition and Physical Activity Behaviors That Lead to Weight Gain," *Journal of Health Psychology* 2019: 135910531985120, https://doi.org/10.1177/1359105319851205.

18   **potential cause for type 2 diabetes** R. S. Surwit, M. S. Schneider, and M. N. Feinglos, "Stress and Diabetes Mellitus," *Diabetes Care* 15, no. 10 (1992): 1413–22, https://doi.org/10.2337/diacare.15.10.1413.

18   **metabolic syndrome** Miroslaw Janczura, Grazyna Bochenek, Roman Nowobilski, Jerzy Dropinski, Katarzyna Kotula-Horowitz, Bartosz Laskowicz, Andrzej Stanisz, Jacek Lelakowski, and Teresa Domagala, "The Relationship of Metabolic Syndrome with Stress, Coronary Heart Disease and Pulmonary Function—An Occupational Cohort-Based Study," *PLOS ONE* 10, no. 8 (2015), https://doi.org/10.1371/journal.pone.0133750.

18   **A 2006 study** Tarani Chandola, Eric Brunner, and Michael Marmot, "Chronic Stress at Work and the Metabolic Syndrome: Prospective Study," *BMJ* 332, no. 7540 (2006): 521–25, https://doi.org/10.1136/bmj.38693.435301.80.

18   **autoimmune conditions have been linked** Chandola, Brunner, and Marmot, "Chronic Stress at Work."

18   **can lead to chronic inflammation** D. S. Bailey, "Burnout Harms Workers' Physical Health through Many Pathways," *Monitor on Psychology* 37, no. 7 (2006): 11, http://www.apa.org/monitor/jun06/burnout.

18   **not in a good way** Armita Golkar, Emilia Johansson, Maki Kasahara, Walter Osika, Aleksander Perski, and Ivanka Savic, "The Influence of Work-Related Chronic Stress on the Regulation of Emotion and on Functional Connectivity in the Brain," *PLOS ONE* 9, no. 9 (2014), https://doi.org/10.1371/journal.pone.0104550.

18   **Your prefrontal cortex thins** Golkar, Johansson, Kasahara, Osika, Perski, and Savic, "Influence of Work-Related Chronic Stress on the Regulation of Emotion."

18   **memory and attention are impacted** Golkar, Johansson, Kasahara, Osika, Perski, and Savic, "Influence of Work-Related Chronic Stress on the Regulation of Emotion."

18   **harder to be creative** Pavlos Deligkaris, Efharis Panagopoulou, Anthony J. Montgomery, and Elvira Masoura, "Job Burnout and Cognitive Functioning: A Systematic Review," *Work & Stress* 28, no. 2 (2014): 107–23, DOI: 10.1080/02678373.2014.909545.

20   **the burnout generation** Anne Helen Petersen, "How Millennials Became the Burnout Generation," BuzzFeed News, August 2, 2020, https://www.buzzfeednews.com/article/annehelenpetersen/millennials-burnout-generation-debt-work.

20   **seeing the "American Dream collapsing"** Jim Tankersley, "American Dream Collapsing for Young Adults, Study Says, as Odds Plunge That Children Will Earn More than Their Parents," *Washington Post*, December 8, 2016, https://www.washingtonpost.com/news/wonk/wp/2016/12/08/american-dream-collapsing-for-young-americans-study-says-finding-plunging-odds-that-children-earn-more-than-their-parents/.

20   **a report on the Blue Cross Blue Shield Health Index** "Two Million Commercially Insured Americans Diagnosed with Major Depression Are Not Seeking Any Treatment," Blue Cross Blue Shield, accessed August 9, 2020, https://www.bcbs.com/the-health-of-america/articles/two-million-commercially-insured-americans-diagnosed-major-depression-not-seeking-treatment.

20   **more of them are dying young** Trust for America's Health and Well Being Trust, *Pain in the Nation: Building a National Resilience Strategy Alcohol and Drug Misuse and Suicide and the Millennial Generation—a Devastating Impact,* 2019.

20   **we lost 36,000 millennials** Jamie Ducharme, "More Millennials Are Dying 'Deaths of Despair,' Report Says," *Time,* June 13, 2019, https://time.com/5606411/millennials-deaths-of-despair/.

20   **it's millennials who lack social support** Minda Zetlin, "Millennials Are the Loneliest Generation, a Survey Shows," Inc.com, September 20, 2019, https://www.inc.com/minda-zetlin/millennials-loneliness-no-friends-friendships-baby-boomers-yougov.html.

Chapter 2

29   **we make more than two hundred decisions** Brian Wansink and Jeffery Sobal, "Mindless Eating: The 200 Daily Food Decisions We Overlook," *Environment and Behavior* 39, no. 1 (January 2007): 106–23, https://doi.org/10.1177/0013916506295573.

31   **half of the recommended intake for fiber** M. K. Hoy and J. D. Goldman, *Fiber Intake of the U.S. Population: What We Eat in America,* National Health and Nutrition Examination Survey 2009–2010, Food Surveys Research Group Dietary Data Brief No. 12, September 2014.

31   **Soluble fiber has been shown** Lisa Brown, Bernard Rosner, Walter W. Willett, and Frank M. Sacks, "Cholesterol-Lowering Effects of Dietary Fiber: A Meta-Analysis," *American Journal of Clinical Nutrition* 69, no. 1 (1999): 30–42, https://doi.org/10.1093/ajcn/69.1.30.

31   **This can help prevent constipation** Jing Yang, "Effect of Dietary Fiber on Constipation: A Meta Analysis," *World Journal of Gastroenterology* 18, no. 48 (2012): 7378, https://doi.org/10.3748/wjg.v18.i48.7378.

31   **95 percent of U.S. adults and kids** Diane Quagliani and Patricia Felt-Gunderson, "Closing America's Fiber Intake Gap," *American Journal of Lifestyle Medicine* 11, no. 1 (2016): 80–85, https://doi.org/10.1177/1559827615588079.

31   **one in ten adults hits the mark** "Only 1 in 10 Adults Get Enough Fruits or Vegetables," Centers for Disease Control and Prevention, November 16, 2017, https://www.cdc.gov/media/releases/2017/p1116-fruit-vegetable-consumption.html.

31   **Weight loss or maintenance** Ru-Yi Huang, Chuan-Chin Huang, Frank B. Hu, and Jorge E. Chavarro, "Vegetarian Diets and Weight Reduction: A Meta-Analysis of Randomized Controlled Trials," *Journal of General Internal Medicine* 31, no. 1 (2015): 109–16, https://doi.org/10.1007/s11606-015-3390-7.

31   **Lower risk of heart disease** Hyunju Kim, Laura E. Caulfield, Vanessa Garcia–Larsen, Lyn M. Steffen, Josef Coresh, and Casey M. Rebholz, "Plant–Based Diets Are Associated with a Lower Risk of Incident Cardiovascular Disease, Cardiovascular Disease Mortality, and All–Cause Mortality in a General Population of Middle–Aged Adults," *Journal of the American Heart Association* 8, no. 16 (2019), https://doi.org/10.1161/jaha.119.012865.

31   **Lower risks for certain types of cancer** Y. Tantamango-Bartley, K. Jaceldo-Siegl, J. Fan, and G. Fraser, "Vegetarian Diets and the Incidence of Cancer in a Low-Risk Population," *Cancer Epidemiology Biomarkers & Prevention* 22, no. 2 (2012): 286–94, https://doi.org/10.1158/1055-9965.epi-12-1060.

31   **Lower rates of cognitive decline** D. Malar and K. Devi, "Dietary Polyphenols for Treatment of Alzheimer's Disease–Future Research and Development," *Current Pharmaceutical Biotechnology* 15, no. 4 (2014): 330–42, https://doi.org/10.2174/1389201015666140813122703.

31   **Lower rates of type 2 diabetes** Ambika Satija, Shilpa N. Bhupathiraju, Eric B. Rimm, Donna Spiegelman, Stephanie E. Chiuve, Lea Borgi, Walter C. Willett, Joann E. Manson, Qi Sun, and Frank B. Hu, "Plant-Based Dietary Patterns and Incidence of Type 2 Diabetes in US Men and Women: Results from Three Prospective Cohort Studies," *PLOS Medicine* 13, no. 6 (2016), https://doi.org/10.1371/journal.pmed.1002039.

33   **2020 Dietary Guidelines for Americans** U.S. Department of Agriculture and U.S. Department of Health and Human Services. *Dietary Guidelines for Americans, 2020-2025.* 9th Edition. December 2020. Available at **DietaryGuidelines.gov**.

33   **undesirable or even toxic results** "Dietary Supplements: What You Need to Know," NIH Office of Dietary Supplements, U.S. Department of Health and Human Services, accessed August 9, 2020, https://ods.od.nih.gov/HealthInformation/DS_WhatYouNeedToKnow.aspx.

35   **They're concentrated sources of phytonutrients** Mauro Serafini and Ilaria Peluso, "Functional Foods for Health: The Interrelated Antioxidant and Anti-Inflammatory Role of Fruits, Vegetables, Herbs, Spices and Cocoa in Humans," *Current Pharmaceutical Design* 22, no. 44 (2017): 6701–15, https://doi.org/10.2174/1381612823666161123094235.

Chapter 3

46   **Research has found** Panagiota Koutsimani, Anthony Montgomery, and Katerina Georganta, "The Relationship between Burnout, Depression, and Anxiety: A Systematic Review and Meta-Analysis," *Frontiers in Psychology* 10 (2019), https://doi.org/10.3389/fpsyg.2019.00284.

46   **In small doses** Francesca Coltrera, "Anxiety: What It Is, What to Do," *Harvard Health Blog,* May 29, 2018, https://www.health.harvard.edu/blog/anxiety-what-it-is-what-to-do-2018060113955.

47   **hormones may even be the reason** "What Is the Link between Women's Hormones and Mood Disorders?" ScienceDaily, December 17, 2007, https://www.sciencedaily.com/releases/2007/12/071212201208.htm.

47   **Premenstrual syndrome** "PMS Relief," Office on Women's Health, U.S. Department of Health and Human Services, March 16, 2018, https://www.womenshealth.gov/menstrual-cycle/premenstrual-syndrome.

47   **PMS can cause moodiness** "PMS Relief."

47   **Here's a quick refresher** "Menstrual Cycle Tool," Office on Women's Health, U.S. Department of Health and Human Services, March 16, 2018, https://www.womenshealth.gov/menstrual-cycle/your-menstrual-cycle.

48   **menopause and the years leading up to it** "Menopause," Office on Women's Health, U.S. Department of Health and Human Services, May 23, 2019, https://www.womenshealth.gov/menopause.

48   **women were at a greater risk** Joyce T. Bromberger and Howard M. Kravitz, "Mood and Menopause: Findings from the Study of Women's Health Across the Nation (SWAN) over 10 Years," *Obstetrics and Gynecology Clinics of North America* 38, no. 3 (2011): 609–25, https://doi.org/10.1016/j.ogc.2011.05.011.

48   **affecting one in nine new moms** "Trends in Postpartum Depressive Symptoms—27 States, 2004, 2008, and 2012," Centers for Disease Control and Prevention, August 1, 2017. https://www.cdc.gov/mmwr/volumes/66/wr/mm6606a1.htm.

48   **Within one day of giving birth** "Postpartum Depression," Office on Women's Health, U.S. Department of Health and Human Services, May 14, 2019, https://www.womenshealth.gov/mental-health/mental-health-conditions/postpartum-depression.

49   **A study published by the** *Journal of Positive Psychology* Calum Neill, Janelle Gerard, and Katherine D. Arbuthnott, "Nature Contact and Mood Benefits: Contact Duration and Mood Type," *Journal of Positive Psychology* 14, no. 6 (2018): 756–67, https://doi.org/10.1080/17439760.2018.15 57242.

49   **Self-transcendence is simply the realization** "What Is Self-Transcendence? Definition and 6 Examples," PositivePsychology.com, May 12, 2020. https://positive psychology.com/self-transcendence/.

49   **Research into the relationship** Rita Berto, "The Role of Nature in Coping with Psycho-physiological Stress: A Literature Review on Restorativeness," *Behavioral Sciences* 4, no. 4 (2014): 394–409, https://doi.org/10.3390/bs4040394.

49   **the gut-brain axis** Emeran A. Mayer, Bruce Naliboff, and Julie Munakata, "The Evolving Neurobiology of Gut Feelings," in *Biological Basis for Mind Body Interactions,* Progress in Brain Research vol. 122 (ScienceDirect: Elsevier, 2000), 195–206, https://doi.org/10.1016/s0079-6123(08)62139-1.

50   **between 200 and 600 million neurons** Emeran A. Mayer, "Gut Feelings: The Emerging Biology of Gut–Brain Communication," *Nature Reviews Neuroscience* 12, no. 8 (2011): 453–66, https://doi.org/10.1038/nrn3071.

50   **enteric nervous system** Meenakshi Rao and Michael D. Gershon, "The Bowel and Beyond: The Enteric Nervous System in Neurological Disorders," *Nature Reviews Gastroenterology & Hepatology* 13, no. 9 (2016): 517–28, https://doi.org/10.1038/nrgastro.2016.107.

50   **reduced "vagal tone"** Sonia Pellissier, Cécile Dantzer, Laurie Mondillon, Candice Trocme, Anne-Sophie Gauchez, Véronique Ducros, Nicolas Mathieu, et al., "Relationship between Vagal Tone, Cortisol, TNF-Alpha, Epinephrine and Negative Affects in Crohn's Disease and Irritable Bowel Syndrome," *PLoS ONE* 9, no. 9 (2014), https://doi.org/10.1371/journal.pone.0105328.

50   **a proven way to stimulate the vagus nerve** Shu-Zhen Wang, Sha Li, Xiao-Yang Xu, Gui-Ping Lin, Li Shao, Yan Zhao, and Ting Huai Wang, "Effect of Slow Abdominal Breathing Combined with Biofeedback on Blood Pressure and Heart Rate Variability in Prehypertension," *Journal of Alternative and Complementary Medicine* 16, no. 10 (2010): 1039–45, https://doi.org/10.1009/acm.2009.0577.

51   **Aromatherapy uses essential oils** Integrative, PDQ, Alternative, and Complementary Therapies Editorial Board, "Aromatherapy with Essential Oils," PDQ Cancer Information Summaries, U.S. National Library of Medicine, March 9, 2007, https://www.ncbi.nlm.nih.gov/books/NBK65820/.

51   **lavender for sleep** Inn Sook Lee and Gyung Joo Lee, "Effects of Lavender Aromatherapy on Insomnia and Depression in Women College Students," *Journal of Korean Academy of Nursing* 36, no. 1 (2006): 136, https://doi.org/10.4040/jkan.2006.36.1.136.

51   **rosemary for focus** O. V. Filiptsova, L. V. Gazzavi-Rogozina, I. A. Timoshyna, O. I. Naboka, Ye. V. Dyomina, and A. V. Ochkur, "The Effect of the Essential Oils of Lavender and Rosemary on the Human Short-Term Memory," *Alexandria Journal of Medicine* 54, no. 1 (2018): 41–44, https://doi.org/10.1016/j.ajme.2017.05.004.

51   **peppermint for energy during exercise** Abbas Meamarbashi and Ali Rajabi, "The Effects of Peppermint on Exercise Performance," *Journal of the International Society of Sports Nutrition* 10, no. 1 (2013), https://doi.org/10.1186/1550-2783-10-15.

51   **which have been shown to boost positive mood** Janice K. Kiecolt-Glaser, Jennifer E. Graham, William B. Malarkey, Kyle Porter, Stanley Lemeshow, and Ronald Glaser, "Olfactory Influences on Mood and Autonomic, Endocrine, and Immune Function," *Psychoneuroendocrinology* 33, no. 3 (2008): 328–39, https://doi.org/10.1016/j.psyneuen.2007.11.015.

51   **has even been shown to reduce anxiety** Mahbubeh Tabatabaeichehr, Fahimeh Rashidi-Fakari, and Hamed Mortazavi, "The Effect of Aromatherapy by Essential Oil of Orange on Anxiety during Labor: A Randomized Clinical Trial," *Iranian Journal of Nursing and Midwifery Research* 20, no. 6 (2015): 661, https://doi.org/10.4103/1735-9066.170001.

51   **other citrus blends** Teruhisa Komori, Ryoichi Fujiwara, Masahiro Tanida, Junichi Nomura, and Mitchel M. Yokoyama, "Effects of Citrus Fragrance on Immune Function and Depressive States," *Neuroimmunomodulation* 2, no. 3 (1995): 174–80, https://doi.org/10.1159/000096889.

52   **trillions of microbes** Gerard Clarke, Roman M. Stilling, Paul J. Kennedy, Catherine Stanton, John F. Cryan, and Timothy G. Dinan, "Minireview: Gut Microbiota: The Neglected Endocrine Organ," *Molecular Endocrinology* 28, no. 8 (2014): 1221–38, https://doi.org/10.1210/me.2014-1108.

52   **beneficial mood-boosting neurotransmitters like GABA** Lucía Diez-Gutiérrez, Leire San Vicente, Luis Javier R. Barrón, María del Carmen Villarán, and María Chávarri, "Gamma-Aminobutyric Acid and Probiotics: Multiple Health Benefits and Their Future in the Global Functional Food and Nutraceuticals Market," *Journal of Functional Foods* 64 (2020): 103669, https://doi.org/10.1016/j.jff.2019.103669.

52   **Nutritional psychiatry examines** Felice N. Jacka, "Nutritional Psychiatry: Where to Next?" *EBioMedicine* 17 (2017): 24–29, https://doi.org/10.1016/j.ebiom.2017.02.020.

52   **Australian researchers are looking** "Our Research," Food and Mood Centre, January 8, 2019, https://foodandmoodcentre.com.au/our-research/.

52 **a small but mighty study** Felice N. Jacka, Adrienne O'Neil, Rachelle Opie, Catherine Itsiopoulos, Sue Cotton, Mohammedreza Mohebbi, David Castle, et al., "A Randomised Controlled Trial of Dietary Improvement for Adults with Major Depression (the 'SMILES' Trial)," *BMC Medicine* 15, no. 1 (2017), https://doi.org/10.1186/s12916-017-0791-y.

53 **Blue Zones** "History of Blue Zones," Blue Zones, February 26, 2019, https://www.bluezones.com/about/history/.

53 **American Gut Project** "American Gut Project," American Gut, accessed August 9, 2020, http://americangut.org/.

53 **related to your risk of depression** Faezeh Saghafian, Hanieh Malmir, Parvane Saneei, Alireza Milajerdi, Bagher Larijani, and Ahmad Esmaillzadeh, "Fruit and Vegetable Consumption and Risk of Depression: Accumulative Evidence from an Updated Systematic Review and Meta-Analysis of Epidemiological Studies," *British Journal of Nutrition* 119, no. 10 (2018): 1087–1101, https://doi.org/10.1017/s0007114518000697.

Chapter 4

61 **Immune cells and tissues are responsible** "How Does the Immune System Work?" InformedHealth.org, U.S. National Library of Medicine, April 23, 2020, https://www.ncbi.nlm.nih.gov/books/NBK279364/.

61 **two types of immunity** "Features of an Immune Response," National Institute of Allergy and Infectious Diseases, U.S. Department of Health and Human Services, accessed August 9, 2020, https://www.niaid.nih.gov/research/immune-response-features.

62 **exercise stimulates certain aspects** David C. Nieman and Laurel M. Wentz, "The Compelling Link between Physical Activity and the Body's Defense System," *Journal of Sport and Health Science* 8, no. 3 (2019): 201–17, https://doi.org/10.1016/j.jshs.2018.09.009.

62 **Every time you exercise** "Exercise and Immunity," Medical Encyclopedia, MedlinePlus, U.S. National Library of Medicine, accessed August 9, 2020. https://medlineplus.gov/ency/article/007165.htm.

62 **a poll by the National Sleep Foundation** "Annual Sleep in America Poll Exploring Connections with Communications Technology Use and Sleep," Sleep Foundation, July 28, 2020, https://www.sleepfoundation.org/media-center/press-release/annual-sleep-america-poll-exploring-connections-communications-technology-use-.

62 **cause levels of an immunoprotective antibody** A. Romero-Martínez, M. Lila, S. Vitoria-Estruch, and L. Moya-Albiol, "High Immunoglobulin A Levels Mediate the Association between High Anger Expression and Low Somatic Symptoms in Intimate Partner Violence Perpetrators," *Journal of Interpersonal Violence* 31, no. 4 (2014): 732–42, https://doi.org/10.1177/0886260514556107.

63 **When we experience a catastrophe or trauma** Glaser, Ronald and J. Kiecolt-Glaser. "How stress damages immune system and health." *Discovery medicine* 5 26 (2005): 165-9. https://www.semanticscholar.org/paper/How-stress-damages-immune-system-and-health.-Glaser-Kiecolt-Glaser/ed66100f4233fed03b78bdababbec814938d1a1c?p2df.

63 **interfere with our immune function** Suzanne C. Segerstrom and Gregory E. Miller, "Psychological Stress and the Human Immune System: A Meta-Analytic Study of 30 Years of Inquiry," *Psychological Bulletin* 130, no. 4 (2004): 601–30, https://doi.org/10.1037/0033-2909.130.4.601.

63 **engage in "friendly fire"** "Too Exhausted to Fight, Immune System May Harm the Body They Are Supposed to Protect," ScienceDaily, June 29, 2015. https://www.sciencedaily.com/releases/2015/06/150629110803.htm.

65 **That adage dates back to 1574** Mark Fischetti, "Fact or Fiction?: Feed a Cold, Starve a Fever," *Scientific American*, January 3, 2014, https://www.scientificamerican.com/article/fact-or-fiction-feed-a-cold/.

Chapter 5

72 **That's called the *doorway effect*** Charles B. Brenner, "Why Walking through a Doorway Makes You Forget," *Scientific American*, December 13, 2011, https://www.scientificamerican.com/article/why-walking-through-doorway-makes-you-forget/.

73 **burnout can alter a person's brain** Alexandra Michel, "Burnout and the Brain," Association for Psychological Science, January 29, 2016, https://www.psychologicalscience.org/observer/burnout-and-the-brain.

73 **burnout impacts cognitive function** P. Deligkaris, E. Panagopoulou, A. J. Montgomery, and E. Masoura, "Job Burnout and Cognitive Functioning: A Systematic Review," *Work & Stress* 28 (2014): 107–123, DOI: 10.1080/02678373.2014.909545

73 **A 2012 review of burnout** Gary Morse, Michelle P. Salyers, Angela L. Rollins, Maria Monroe-Devita, and Corey Pfahler, "Burnout in Mental Health Services: A Review of the Problem and Its Remediation," *Administration and Policy in Mental Health and Mental Health Services Research* 39, no. 5 (2011): 341–52, https://doi.org/10.1007/s10488-011-0352-1.

76 **there are two types** Yoshihito Shigihara, Masaaki Tanaka, Akira Ishii, Etsuko Kanai, Masami Funakura, and Yasuyoshi Watanabe, "Two Types of Mental Fatigue Affect

Spontaneous Oscillatory Brain Activities in Different Ways," *Behavioral and Brain Functions* 9, no. 1 (2013): 2, https://doi .org/10.1186/1744-9081-9-2.

76   **cognitive signs of burnout** Krystyna Golonka, Justyna Mojsa-Kaja, Magda Gawlowska, and Katarzyna Popiel, "Cognitive Impairments in Occupational Burnout— Error Processing and Its Indices of Reactive and Proactive Control," *Frontiers in Psychology* 8 (2017), https://doi.org/ 10.3389/fpsyg.2017.00676.

76   **Symptoms of ADHD vary** "Attention-Deficit/ Hyperactivity Disorder," National Institute of Mental Health, U.S. Department of Health and Human Services, accessed August 9, 2020, https://www.nimh.nih.gov/health/topics/ attention-deficit-hyperactivity-disorder-adhd/index.shtml.

77   **According to a groundbreaking study** M. Virtanen, A. Singh-Manoux, J. E. Ferrie, D. Gimeno, M. G. Marmot, M. Elovainio, M. Jokela, J. Vahtera, and M. Kivimaki, "Long Working Hours and Cognitive Function: The Whitehall II Study," *American Journal of Epidemiology* 169, no. 5 (2008): 596–605, https://doi.org/10.1093/aje/kwn382.

77   **A report from the CDC** National Institute for Occupational Safety and Health, *Overtime and Extended Work Shifts: Recent Findings on Illnesses, Injuries and Health Behaviors*, Centers for Disease Control and Prevention, June 6, 2014, https://www.cdc.gov/niosh/docs/2004-143/ default.html.

78   **Decision fatigue is why** Adam F. Stewart, Donna M. Ferriero, S. Andrew Josephson, Daniel H. Lowenstein, Robert O. Messing, Jorge R. Oksenberg, S. Claiborne Johnston, and Stephen L. Hauser, "Fighting Decision Fatigue," *Annals of Neurology* 71, no. 1 (2012), https://doi.org/10.1002/ana.23531.

78   **Kahl, a New York art director** Megan Willett, "This Woman Has Worn the Same Outfit to Work Every Single Day for the Past 3 Years," *Business Insider*, April 24, 2015, https://www.businessinsider.com/ woman-wears-same-work-outfit-matilda-kahl-2015-4.

79   **Research at Rice University in 2014** Katharine Ridgway O'Brien, "Just Saying 'No': An Examination of Gender Differences in the Ability to Decline Requests in the Workplace," Rice Scholarship Home, May 1, 2014, https:// scholarship.rice.edu/handle/1911/77421.

79   **Researchers in 2011 found** Vanessa M. Patrick and Henrik Hagtvedt, "'I Don't' versus 'I Can't': When Empowered Refusal Motivates Goal-Directed Behavior," *Journal of Consumer Research* 39, no. 2 (2012): 371–81, https://doi.org/ 10.1086/663212.

80   **Multitasking actually impairs productivity** "Multitasking: Switching Costs," American Psychological Association, accessed August 9, 2020, https://www.apa .org/research/action/multitask.

80   **endurance exercise offers your brain** Cell Press, "Molecule Produced during Exercise Boosts Brain Health," EurekAlert!, October 10, 2013, https://www.eurekalert.org/ pub_releases/2013-10/cp-mpd100313.php.

81   **we help our brain stay sharp** "Learning New Skills Keeps an Aging Mind Sharp," Association for Psychological Science, October 21, 2013, http://www.psychologicalscience. org/index.php/news/releases/learning-new-skills-keeps -an-aging-mind-sharp.html.

81   **gives us a little hit of dopamine** Stephen Hartley, "Dopamine, Smartphones & You: A Battle for Your Time," Science in the News, Harvard University, February 27, 2019, http://sitn.hms.harvard.edu/flash/2018/ dopamine-smartphones-battle-time/.

81   **which can help prevent cognitive decline** William Harms, "AAAS 2014: Loneliness Is a Major Health Risk for Older Adults," University of Chicago News, accessed August 9, 2020, http://news.uchicago.edu/article/2014/02/16/ aaas-2014-loneliness-major-health-risk-older-adults.

81   **Meditation changes your brain patterns** Joshua Gowin, "Brain Scans Show How Meditation Improves Mental Focus," Psychology Today, April 20, 2012, https://www. psychologytoday.com/us/blog/you-illuminated/201204/ brain-scans-show-how-meditation-improves-mental-focus.

81   **A 2019 study found** Yanli Lin, William D. Eckerle, Ling W. Peng, and Jason S. Moser, "On Variation in Mindfulness Training: A Multimodal Study of Brief Open Monitoring Meditation on Error Monitoring," *Brain Sciences* 9, no. 9 (2019): 226, https://doi.org/10.3390/brainsci9090226

81   **train your brain to stay focused on a task** Joan P. Pozuelos, Bethan R. Mead, M. Rosario Rueda, and Peter Malinowski, "Short-Term Mindful Breath Awareness Training Improves Inhibitory Control and Response Monitoring," in *Meditation*, Progress in Brain Research vol. 244 (ScienceDirect: Elsevier, 2019), 137–63, https://www.science direct.com/science/article/pii/S0079612318301584?via=ihub.

81   **help you manage stress** Jose L. Herrero, Simon Khuvis, Erin Yeagle, Moran Cerf, and Ashesh D. Mehta, "Breathing above the Brain Stem: Volitional Control and Attentional Modulation in Humans," *Journal of Neurophysiology* 119, no. 1 (2018):145–59, https://journals. physiology.org/doi/full/10.1152/jn.00551.2017.

81   **Research from 2010** Nicole Lovato and Leon Lack, "The Effects of Napping on Cognitive Functioning," in *Human Sleep and Cognition*, Progress in Brain Research vol. 185, (ScienceDirect: Elsevier, 2010), 155–66, https://doi.org/10.1016/ b978-0-444-53702-7.00009-9.

83   **influence a number of biological systems** Katherine H. M. Cox and Andrew Scholey, "Polyphenols for Brain and Cognitive Health," in *Recent Advances in Polyphenol*

Research, eds. Kumi Yoshida, Véronique Cheynier, and Stéphane Quideau (Wiley Online Library: John Wiley & Sons: 2016), https://onlinelibrary.wiley.com/doi/abs/10.1002/9781118883303.ch12.

83 **help improve memory issues as we age** Marshall G. Miller, Derek A. Hamilton, James A. Joseph, and Barbara Shukitt-Hale, "Dietary Blueberry Improves Cognition among Older Adults in a Randomized, Double-Blind, Placebo-Controlled Trial," *European Journal of Nutrition* 57, no. 3 (2017): 1169–80, https://doi.org/10.1007/s00394-017-1400-8.

83 **they can also delay cognitive decline** Elizabeth E. Devore, Jae Hee Kang, Monique M. B. Breteler, and Francine Grodstein, "Dietary Intakes of Berries and Flavonoids in Relation to Cognitive Decline," *Annals of Neurology* 72, no. 1 (2012): 135–43, https://doi.org/10.1002/ana.23594.

83 **access regions involved in learning** Devore, Kang, Breteler, and Grodstein. "Dietary Intakes of Berries and Flavonoids."

83 **grapes may support brain health** J. K. Lee, N. Torsyan, and D. H. Silverman, "Examining the Impact of Grape Consumption on Brain Metabolism and Cognitive Function in Patients with Mild Decline in Cognition: A Double-Blinded Placebo-Controlled Pilot Study," *Experimental Gerontology* 87 (Pt A):121–28.

83 **Dark chocolate also provides flavonoids** Astrid Nehlig, "The Neuroprotective Effects of Cocoa Flavanol and Its Influence on Cognitive Performance," *British Journal of Clinical Pharmacology* 75, no. 3 (2013): 716–27, https://doi.org/10.1111/j.1365-2125.2012.04378.x.

83 **Deficiencies of certain essential nutrients** Michal Novotný, Blanka Klimova, and Martin Valis, "Microbiome and Cognitive Impairment: Can Any Diets Influence Learning Processes in a Positive Way?" *Frontiers in Aging Neuroscience* 11 (2019), https://doi.org/10.3389/fnagi.2019.00170.

83 **While the jury is still out** Serena Verdi, Matthew A. Jackson, Michelle Beaumont, Ruth C. E. Bowyer, Jordana T. Bell, Tim D. Spector, and Claire J. Steves, "An Investigation into Physical Frailty as a Link between the Gut Microbiome and Cognitive Health," *Frontiers in Aging Neuroscience* 10 (2018), https://doi.org/10.3389/fnagi.2018.00398.

83 **researchers studied the diets** Esme Fuller-Thomson, Z. Saab, K. M. Davison, S. Lamson Lin, V. Taler, K. Kobayashi, and H. Tong, "Nutrition, Immigration and Health Determinants Are Linked to Verbal Fluency among Anglophone Adults in the Canadian Longitudinal Study on Aging (CLSA)," *Journal of Nutrition, Health & Aging* 24, no. 6 (2020): 672–80, https://doi.org/10.1007/s12603-020-1402-8.

Chapter 6

90 **a survey by the Better Sleep Council** "Not Tonight, Honey." Better Sleep Council | Start every day with a good night's sleep, February 24, 2021. https://bettersleep.org/research/sleep-surveys/survey-americans-crave-sleep-more-than-sex/.

90 **the main symptom of sleep deprivation** "Sleep Deprivation Fact Sheet," American Academy of Sleep Medicine, 2008.

92 **Shifting hormones during and after pregnancy** Peter F. Schnatz, Sabrina Kum Whitehurst, and David M. O'Sullivan, "Sexual Dysfunction, Depression, and Anxiety among Patients of an Inner-City Menopause Clinic," *Journal of Women's Health* 19, no. 10 (2010): 1843–49, https://doi.org/10.1089/jwh.2009.1800.

92 **A 2019 study of postmenopausal women** David A. Kalmbach, Sheryl A. Kingsberg, Thomas Roth, Philip Cheng, Cynthia Fellman-Couture, and Christopher L. Drake, "Sexual Function and Distress in Postmenopausal Women with Chronic Insomnia: Exploring the Role of Stress Dysregulation," *Nature and Science of Sleep* 11 (2019): 141–53, https://doi.org/10.2147/nss.s213941.

92 **researchers have floated the idea** David A. Kalmbach, J. Todd Arnedt, Vivek Pillai, and Jeffrey A. Ciesla, "The Impact of Sleep on Female Sexual Response and Behavior: A Pilot Study," *Journal of Sexual Medicine* 12, no. 5 (2015): 1221–32, https://doi.org/10.1111/jsm.12858.

92 **Women's Health Initiative observational study** Juliana M. Kling, Joann E. Manson, Michelle J. Naughton, M'Hamed Temkit, Shannon D. Sullivan, Emily W. Gower, Lauren Hale, Julie C. Weitlauf, Sara Nowakowski, and Carolyn J. Crandall, "Association of Sleep Disturbance and Sexual Function in Postmenopausal Women," *Menopause* 24, no. 6 (2017): 604–12, https://doi.org/10.1097/gme.0000000000000824.

92 **sex before bed could help** Amy Khodr, Caroline Awada, Massoot Mohammed, and Reabal Najjar, "Bump and Sleep: How Sexual Intercourse Can Improve Sleep of Women with Insomnia," University of Ottawa research poster, November 26, 2016, https://ruor.uottawa.ca/handle/10393/35554.

93 **closely associated with burnout** Arnaud Metlaine, Fabien Sauvet, Danielle Gomez-Merino, Maxime Elbaz, Jean Yves Delafosse, Damien Leger, and Mounir Chennaoui, "Association between Insomnia Symptoms, Job Strain and Burnout Syndrome: A Cross-Sectional Survey of 1300 Financial Workers," *BMJ Open* 7, no. 1 (2017), https://doi.org/10.1136/bmjopen-2016-012816.

93 **a 2020 poll by the National Sleep Foundation** "The National Sleep Foundation's 2020 Sleep in America Poll Shows Alarming Level of Sleepiness and Low Levels of

Action," Sleep Foundation, July 28, 2020, https://www
.sleepfoundation.org/press-release/nsfs-2020-sleep
-america-poll-shows-alarming-sleepiness-and-low-action.

93   **your memory suffers** "Why Lack of Sleep Is
Bad for Your Health," NHS Choices, National Health
Service (UK), accessed August 9, 2020, https://
www.nhs.uk/live-well/sleep-and-tiredness/
why-lack-of-sleep-is-bad-for-your-health/.

93   **A 2013 study out of Sweden** "Study Reveals
the Face of Sleep Deprivation," American Academy
of Sleep Medicine, March 13, 2018, https://aasm.org/
study-reveals-the-face-of-sleep-deprivation/.

93   **Sleep also impacts two hormones** Erika W. Hagen,
Samuel J. Starke, and Paul E. Peppard, "The Association
between Sleep Duration and Leptin, Ghrelin, and
Adiponectin among Children and Adolescents," *Current
Sleep Medicine Reports* 1, no. 4 (2015): 185–94, https://doi
.org/10.1007/s40675-015-0025-9.

94   **may cause a chemical shift** Erin C. Hanlon, Esra
Tasali, Rachel Leproult, Kara L. Stuhr, Elizabeth Doncheck,
Harriet De Wit, Cecilia J. Hillard, and Eve Van Cauter, "Sleep
Restriction Enhances the Daily Rhythm of Circulating Levels
of Endocannabinoid 2-Arachidonoylglycerol," *Sleep* 39, no. 3
(2016): 653–64, https://doi.org/10.5665/sleep.5546.

94   **A lengthy study found** "Sleeping Less Linked to
Weight Gain," ScienceDaily, May 29, 2006, https://www
.sciencedaily.com/releases/2006/05/060529082903.htm.

94   **A review of thirty-six studies** Sanjay R. Patel and
Frank B. Hu, "Short Sleep Duration and Weight Gain: A
Systematic Review," *Obesity* 16, no. 3 (2008): 643–53, https://
doi.org/10.1038/oby.2007.118.

94   **A 2019 study involving women** Chia-Lun Yang,
Jerry Schnepp, and Robin Tucker, "Increased Hunger, Food
Cravings, Food Reward, and Portion Size Selection after
Sleep Curtailment in Women without Obesity," *Nutrients* 11,
no. 3 (2019): 663, https://doi.org/10.3390/nu11030663.

94   **sleep disturbances are a red flag** Michele Lastella,
Grace E. Vincent, Rob Duffield, Gregory D. Roach, Shona L.
Halson, Luke J. Heales, and Charli Sargent, "Can Sleep Be
Used as an Indicator of Overreaching and Overtraining in
Athletes?" *Frontiers in Physiology* 9 (2018), https://doi.org/
10.3389/fphys.2018.00436.

94   **women experience sleep disorders** American
Academy of Sleep Medicine, "Study Finds That Sleep
Disorders Affect Men and Women Differently," EurekAlert!,
May 22, 2017, https://www.eurekalert.org/pub_
releases/2017-05/aaos-sft052217.php.

94   **the CDC reported in 2013** "QuickStats: Percentage of
Adults Who Often Felt Very Tired or Exhausted in the Past
3 Months, by Sex and Age Group—National Health Interview
Survey, United States, 2010–2011," Centers for Disease
Control and Prevention, accessed August 9, 2020, https://
www.cdc.gov/mmwr/preview/mmwrhtml/mm6214a5.
htm?s_cid=mm6214a5_w.

95   **A 2019 survey from Common Sense Media** Michael
Robb, "Tweens, Teens, and Phones: What Our 2019 Research
Reveals," Common Sense Media, October 29, 2019, https://
www.commonsensemedia.org/blog/tweens-teens-and
-phones-what-our-2019-research-reveals.

96   **alcohol can impair your sleep quality** "Alcohol and
Sleep," Sleep Foundation, July 28, 2020, https://www
.sleepfoundation.org/articles/how-alcohol-affects
-quality-and-quantity-sleep.

96   **caffeine has a half-life** Institute of Medicine (U.S.)
Committee on Military Nutrition Research, "Pharmacology
of Caffeine," in *Caffeine for the Sustainment of Mental Task
Performance: Formulations for Military Operations*, U.S.
National Library of Medicine, 2001, https://www.ncbi.nlm
.nih.gov/books/NBK223808/.

96   **Those harsh artificial lights** Christine Blume, Corrado
Garbazza, and Manuel Spitschan, "Effects of Light on
Human Circadian Rhythms, Sleep and Mood," *Somnologie:
Schlafforschung und Schlafmedizin* [Somnology: Sleep
Research and Sleep Medicine] 23, no. 3 (2019): 147–56,
https://www.ncbi.nlm.nih.gov/pmc/articles/PMC6751071/.

97   **One 2014 study of Japanese women** Ryoko Katagiri,
Keiko Asakura, Satomi Kobayashi, Hitomi Suga, and
Satoshi Sasaki, "Low Intake of Vegetables, High Intake of
Confectionary, and Unhealthy Eating Habits Are Associated
with Poor Sleep Quality among Middle-Aged Female
Japanese Workers," *Journal of Occupational Health* 56, no. 5
(2014): 359–68, https://doi.org/10.1539/joh.14-0051-oa.

97   **spicy foods can disrupt sleep** Stephen J. Edwards,
Iain M. Montgomery, Eric Q. Colquhoun, Jo E. Jordan,
and Michael G. Clark, "Spicy Meal Disturbs Sleep: An
Effect of Thermoregulation?" *International Journal of
Psychophysiology* 13, no. 2 (1992): 97–100, https://doi.org/
10.1016/0167-8760(92)90048-g.

97   **according to a 2007 review** Timothy Roehrs and
Thomas Roth, "Caffeine: Sleep and Daytime Sleepiness,"
Sleep Medicine Reviews 12, no. 2 (2008): 153–62, https://doi
.org/10.1016/j.smrv.2007.07.004.

97   **A 2009 study compared the effects** Julie Carrier,
Jean Paquet, Marta Fernandez-Bolanos, Laurence Girouard,
Joanie Roy, Brahim Selmaoui, and Daniel Filipini, "Effects of
Caffeine on Daytime Recovery Sleep: A Double Challenge
to the Sleep–Wake Cycle in Aging," *Sleep Medicine* 10, no. 9
(2009): 1016–24, https://doi.org/10.1016/j.sleep.2009.01.001.

98   Chamomile tea Janmejai K. Srivastava, Eswar Shankar, and Sanjay Gupta, "Chamomile: A Herbal Medicine of the Past with a Bright Future (Review)," *Molecular Medicine Reports* 3, no. 6 (2010): 895–901, https://doi.org/10.3892/mmr.2010.377.

99   lactucin to induce sleep Hae Dun Kim, Ki-Bae Hong, Dong Ouk Noh, and Hyung Joo Suh, "Sleep-Inducing Effect of Lettuce (*Lactuca sativa*) Varieties on Pentobarbital-Induced Sleep," *Food Science and Biotechnology* 26, no. 3 (2017): 807–14, https://doi.org/10.1007/s10068-017-0107-1.

101   it could impact your mood A. Coppen, E. G. Eccleston, and M. Peet, "Total and Free Tryptophan Concentration in the Plasma of Depressive Patients," *Lancet* 302, no. 7820 (1973): 60–63, https://doi.org/10.1016/s0140-6736(73)93259-5.

101   boosting the hormones that regulate R. Bravo, S. Matito, J. Cubero, S. D. Paredes, L. Franco, M. Rivero, A. B. Rodríguez, and C. Barriga, "Tryptophan-Enriched Cereal Intake Improves Nocturnal Sleep, Melatonin, Serotonin, and Total Antioxidant Capacity Levels and Mood in Elderly Humans," *Age* 35, no. 4 (2012): 1277–85, https://doi.org/10.1007/s11357-012-9419-5.

101   high-carb meals have a roundabout way Bonnie Spring, "Recent Research on the Behavioral Effects of Tryptophan and Carbohydrate," *Nutrition and Health* 3, no. 1–2 (1984): 55–67, https://doi.org/10.1177/026010608400300204.

Chapter 7

158   bioactive compounds in peppermint Diane L. McKay and Jeffrey B. Blumberg, "A Review of the Bioactivity and Potential Health Benefits of Peppermint Tea (*Mentha piperita* L.)," *Phytotherapy Research* 20, no. 8 (2006): 619–33, https://doi.org/10.1002/ptr.1936.

158   improve sleep quality Sahar Hamzeh, Roya Safari-Faramani, and Alireza Khatony, "Effects of Aromatherapy with Lavender and Peppermint Essential Oils on the Sleep Quality of Cancer Patients: A Randomized Controlled Trial," *Evidence-Based Complementary and Alternative Medicine* 2020 (2020): 1–7, https://doi.org/10.1155/2020/7480204.

158   Tart cherries contain naturally occurring melatonin Glyn Howatson, Phillip G. Bell, Jamie Tallent, Benita Middleton, Malachy P. McHugh, and Jason Ellis, "Effect of Tart Cherry Juice (*Prunus cerasus*) on Melatonin Levels and Enhanced Sleep Quality," *European Journal of Nutrition* 51, no. 8 (2011): 909–16, https://doi.org/10.1007/s00394-011-0263-7.

160   a compound in lavender called linalool Hiroki Harada, Hideki Kashiwadani, Yuichi Kanmura, and Tomoyuki Kuwaki, "Linalool Odor-Induced Anxiolytic Effects in Mice," *Frontiers in Behavioral Neuroscience* 12 (2018), https://doi.org/10.3389/fnbeh.2018.00241.

160   a compound in lavender called linalool Peir Hossein Koulivand, Maryam Khaleghi Ghadiri, and Ali Gorji, "Lavender and the Nervous System," *Evidence-Based Complementary and Alternative Medicine* 2013 (2013): 1–10, https://doi.org/10.1155/2013/681304.

Appendix 1

223   anti-inflammatory response in immune cells "Fiber in Food Calms Angry Immune Cells," Futurity, October 12, 2010, https://www.futurity.org/fiber-in-food-calms-angry-immune-cells/.

225   Folate plays a role A. L. Miller, "The Methylation, Neurotransmitter, and Antioxidant Connections between Folate and Depression," *Alternative Medicine Review* 13, no. 3 (2008): 216–26.

225   A deficiency in folate levels S. N. Young, "Folate and Depression—a Neglected Problem," *Journal of Psychiatry and Neuroscience* 32, no. 2. (2007): 80–82.

225   Folate shortages are linked E. H. Reynolds, "Folic Acid, Ageing, Depression, and Dementia," *BMJ* 324, no. 7352 (2002): 1512–15. https://doi.org/10.1136/bmj.324.7352.1512.

225   Folate is crucial for cell growth S. J. Duthie, "Folic Acid Deficiency and Cancer: Mechanisms of DNA Instability," *British Medical Bulletin* 55, no. 3 (1999): 578–92, https://doi.org/10.1258/0007142991902646.

225   A B$_6$ deficiency will impact immune function Bingjun Qian, Shanqi Shen, Jianhua Zhang, and Pu Jing, "Effects of Vitamin B6 Deficiency on the Composition and Functional Potential of T Cell Populations," *Journal of Immunology Research* 2017 (2017): 1–12, https://doi.org/10.1155/2017/2197975.

225   A deficiency is linked to memory loss David Kennedy, "B Vitamins and the Brain: Mechanisms, Dose and Efficacy—a Review," *Nutrients* 8, no. 2 (2016): 68, https://doi.org/10.3390/nu8020068.

225   Vitamin B$_{12}$ is believed to influence melatonin G. Mayer, "Effects of Vitamin B12 on Performance and Circadian Rhythm in Normal Subjects," *Neuropsychopharmacology* 15, no. 5 (1996): 456–64, https://doi.org/10.1016/s0893-133x(96)00055-3.

226   Choline is a B-vitamin-like nutrient "Choline," NIH Office of Dietary Supplements, U.S. Department of Health and Human Services, accessed August 17, 2020, https://ods.od.nih.gov/factsheets/Choline-HealthProfessional/.

226 **choline synthesis is linked to estrogen** Steven H. Zeisel and Marie A. Caudill, "Choline," *Advances in Nutrition* 1, no. 1 (2010): 46–48, https://doi.org/10.3945/an.110.1010.

226 **Consuming choline has been studied** "Essential Nutrient May Help Fight Alzheimer's across Generations," ScienceDaily, January 8, 2019, https://www.sciencedaily.com/releases/2019/01/190108084424.htm.

226 **white blood cells require vitamin C** A. Ströhle and A. Hahn, "Vitamin C und Immunfunktion" [Vitamin C and immune function] *Medizinische Monatsschrift für Pharmazeuten* 32, no. 2 (2009): 49–56.

226 **Your adrenal glands require it** Michael H. Hooper, Anitra Carr, and Paul E. Marik, "The Adrenal-Vitamin C Axis: From Fish to Guinea Pigs and Primates," *Critical Care* 23, no. 1 (2019), https://doi.org/10.1186/s13054-019-2332-x.

226 **when you're sleep-deprived** L. A. Olayaki, O. S. Sulaiman, and N. B. Anoba, "Vitamin C Prevents Sleep Deprivation–Induced Elevation in Cortisol and Lipid Peroxidation in the Rat Plasma," *Nigerian Journal of Physiological Sciences* 30, no. 1–2, (2015): 5–9.

226 **Vitamin C functions as an antioxidant** Fiona E. Harrison and James M. May, "Vitamin C Function in the Brain: Vital Role of the Ascorbate Transporter SVCT2," *Free Radical Biology and Medicine* 46, no. 6 (2009): 719–30, https://doi.org/10.1016/j.freeradbiomed.2008.12.018.

226 **protecting your brain from inflammation** Stuart Bennett, Melissa M. Grant, and Sarah Aldred, "Oxidative Stress in Vascular Dementia and Alzheimer's Disease. A Common Pathology," *Journal of Alzheimer's Disease* 17, no. 2 (2008): 245–57, https://doi.org/10.3233/jad-2009-1041.

226 **It protects your intestinal and other linings** Zhiyi Huang, Yu Liu, Guangying Qi, David Brand, and Song Zheng, "Role of Vitamin A in the Immune System," *Journal of Clinical Medicine* 7, no. 9 (2018): 258, https://doi.org/10.3390/jcm7090258.

226 **Vitamin A serves as a signaling molecule** Christopher R. Olson and Claudio V. Mello, "Significance of Vitamin A to Brain Function, Behavior and Learning," *Molecular Nutrition & Food Research* 54, no. 4 (2010): 489–95, https://doi.org/10.1002/mnfr.200900246.

227 **D_3 is more effective** Laura Tripkovic, Helen Lambert, Kathryn Hart, Colin P. Smith, Giselda Bucca, Simon Penson, Gemma Chope, et al., "Comparison of Vitamin D2 and Vitamin D3 Supplementation in Raising Serum 25-Hydroxyvitamin D Status: A Systematic Review and Meta-Analysis," *American Journal of Clinical Nutrition* 95, no. 6 (2012): 1357–64, https://doi.org/10.3945/ajcn.111.031070.

227 **people with depression who receive vitamin D supplements** Sue Penckofer, Joanne Kouba, Mary Byrn, and Carol Estwing Ferrans, "Vitamin D and Depression: Where Is All the Sunshine?" *Issues in Mental Health Nursing* 31, no. 6 (2010): 385–93, https://doi.org/10.3109/01612840903437657.

227 **deficiency can impair cognitive function** Phoebe E. Mayne and Thomas H. J. Burne, "Vitamin D in Synaptic Plasticity, Cognitive Function, and Neuropsychiatric Illness," *Trends in Neurosciences* 42, no. 4 (2019): 293–306, https://doi.org/10.1016/j.tins.2019.01.003.

227 **Low vitamin D negatively affects several aspects** Qi Gao, Tingyan Kou, Bin Zhuang, Yangyang Ren, Xue Dong, and Qiuzhen Wang, "The Association between Vitamin D Deficiency and Sleep Disorders: A Systematic Review and Meta-Analysis," *Nutrients* 10, no. 10 (2018): 1395, https://doi.org/10.3390/nu10101395.

227 **It helps your cells** "Vitamin E," NIH Office of Dietary Supplements, U.S. Department of Health and Human Services, accessed August 17, 2020, https://ods.od.nih.gov/factsheets/VitaminE-HealthProfessional/.

227 **vitamin E acts as an antioxidant** Giorgio Fata, Peter Weber, and M. Mohajeri, "Effects of Vitamin E on Cognitive Performance during Ageing and in Alzheimer's Disease," *Nutrients* 6, no. 12 (2014): 5453–72, https://doi.org/10.3390/nu6125453.

228 **immune and inflammatory responses mediated by T cells** Nazli Namazi, Bagher Larijani, and Leila Azadbakht, "Vitamin K and the Immune System," in *Nutrition and Immunity*, eds. Maryam Mahmoudi and Nima Rezaei (SpringerLink: Springer, 2019), 75–79, https://doi.org/10.1007/978-3-030-16073-9_4.

228 **The mineral can become imbalanced in brain cells** Charlene Supnet and Ilya Bezprozvanny, "The Dysregulation of Intracellular Calcium in Alzheimer Disease," *Cell Calcium* 47, no. 2 (2010): 183–89, https://doi.org/10.1016/j.ceca.2009.12.014.

228 **That's where vitamin K comes in** Ludovico Alisi, Roberta Cao, Cristina de Angelis, Arturo Cafolla, Francesca Caramia, Gaia Cartocci, Aloisa Librando, and Marco Fiorelli, "The Relationships between Vitamin K and Cognition: A Review of Current Evidence," *Frontiers in Neurology* 10 (2019), https://doi.org/10.3389/fneur.2019.00239.

228 **plays a crucial role in managing PMS** "Calcium," NIH Office of Dietary Supplements, U.S. Department of Health and Human Services, accessed August 17, 2020, https://ods.od.nih.gov/factsheets/Calcium-HealthProfessional/.

228 **(along with vitamin D)** Elizabeth R. Bertone-Johnson, Susan E. Hankinson, Adrianne Bendich, Susan R. Johnson, Walter C. Willett, and Joann E. Manson, "Calcium and Vitamin D Intake and Risk of Incident Premenstrual Syndrome," *Archives of Internal Medicine* 165, no. 11 (2005): 1246, https://doi.org/10.1001/archinte.165.11.1246.

228   low intake of calcium Yun-Jung Bae and Soon-Kyung Kim, "Low Dietary Calcium Is Associated with Self-Rated Depression in Middle-Aged Korean Women," *Nutrition Research and Practice* 6, no. 6 (2012): 527, https://doi.org/10.4162/nrp.2012.6.6.527.

228   Calcium plays a role in brain health Pietro Gareri, Rosario Mattace, Felice Nava, and Giovambattista de Sarro, "Role of Calcium in Brain Aging," *General Pharmacology: The Vascular System* 26, no. 8 (1995): 1651–57, https://doi.org/10.1016/0306-3623(95)00043-7.

228   Deficiencies are linked to trouble falling asleep Michael A. Grandner, Nicholas Jackson, Jason R. Gerstner, and Kristen L. Knutson, "Sleep Symptoms Associated with Intake of Specific Dietary Nutrients," *Journal of Sleep Research* 23, no. 1 (2013): 22–34, https://doi.org/10.1111/jsr.12084.

228   shown to help depression George A. Eby and Karen L. Eby, "Magnesium for Treatment-Resistant Depression: A Review and Hypothesis," *Medical Hypotheses* 74, no. 4 (2010): 649–60, https://doi.org/10.1016/j.mehy.2009.10.051.

228   magnesium (with vitamin B$_6$) can improve PMS symptoms N. Fathizadeh, E. Ebrahimi, M. Valiani, N. Tavakoli, and M. H. Yar, "Evaluating the Effect of Magnesium and Magnesium Plus Vitamin B6 Supplement on the Severity of Premenstrual Syndrome," *Iranian Journal of Nursing and Midwifery Research* 15, suppl. 1 (2010): 401–5.

228   magnesium helps control the smooth muscle Institute of Medicine (U.S.) Committee on Nutrition, Trauma, and the Brain, "Magnesium," in *Nutrition and Traumatic Brain Injury: Improving Acute and Subacute Health Outcomes in Military Personnel*, eds. J. Erdman, M. Oria, and L. Pillsbury (Washington, D.C.: National Academies Press, 2011), https://www.ncbi.nlm.nih.gov/books/NBK209305/

228   lower levels of this essential mineral Anna Kirkland, Gabrielle Sarlo, and Kathleen Holton, "The Role of Magnesium in Neurological Disorders," *Nutrients* 10, no. 6 (2018): 730, https://doi.org/10.3390/nu10060730.

229   Anemia (iron deficiency) causes symptoms T. S. Sathyanarayana Rao, M. R. Asha, B. N. Ramesh, and K. S. Jagannatha Rao, "Understanding Nutrition, Depression and Mental Illnesses," *Indian Journal of Psychiatry* 50, no. 2 (2008): 77, https://doi.org/10.4103/0019-5545.42391.

229   The proteins found in iron Sonal Agrawal, Kiersten L. Berggren, Eileen Marks, and Jonathan H. Fox, "Impact of High Iron Intake on Cognition and Neurodegeneration in Humans and in Animal Models: A Systematic Review," *Nutrition Reviews* 75, no. 6 (2017): 456–70, https://doi.org/10.1093/nutrit/nux015.

229   Anemia deprives your body—and brain Laura E. Murray-Kolb, "Iron and Brain Functions," *Current Opinion in Clinical Nutrition and Metabolic Care* 16, no. 6 (2013): 703–7, https://doi.org/10.1097/mco.0b013e3283653ef8.

229   both your innate and your adaptive immune functions Bobby J. Cherayil, "Iron and Immunity: Immunological Consequences of Iron Deficiency and Overload," *Archivum Immunologiae et Therapiae Experimentalis* 58, no. 6 (2010): 407–15, https://doi.org/10.1007/s00005-010-0095-9.

229   When you have healthy levels Roberta J. Ward, Robert R. Crichton, Deanna L. Taylor, Laura Della Corte, Surjit K. Srai, and David T. Dexter, "Iron and the Immune System," *Journal of Neural Transmission* 118, no. 3 (2010): 315–28, https://doi.org/10.1007/s00702-010-0479-3.

229   While your immune system needs copper S. S. Percival, "Copper and Immunity," *American Journal of Clinical Nutrition* 67, no. 5 (1998): 1064S–68S https://doi.org/10.1093/ajcn/67.5.1064s.

229   manages immune cell signals Inga Wessels, Martina Maywald, and Lothar Rink, "Zinc as a Gatekeeper of Immune Function," *Nutrients* 9, no. 12 (2017): 1286, https://doi.org/10.3390/nu9121286.

229   Deficiency of this mineral can cause symptoms Michael Hambidge, "Human Zinc Deficiency," *Journal of Nutrition* 130, no. 5 (2000): 1344S–49S, https://doi.org/10.1093/jn/130.5.1344s.

229   depression, ADHD, difficulties with learning and memory Meihua Piao, Xiaoqiang Cong, Ying Lu, Chunsheng Feng, and Pengfei Ge, "The Role of Zinc in Mood Disorders," *Neuropsychiatry* 7, no. 4 (2018), https://doi.org/10.4172/neuropsychiatry.1000225.

230   may shorten the duration of colds Harri Hemilä, "Zinc Lozenges and the Common Cold: A Meta-Analysis Comparing Zinc Acetate and Zinc Gluconate, and the Role of Zinc Dosage," *JRSM Open* 8, no. 5 (2017): 205427041769429, https://doi.org/10.1177/2054270417694291.

230   manages your immune system's inflammatory responses "Zinc Helps against Infection by Tapping Brakes in Immune Response," ScienceDaily, February 7, 2013, https://www.sciencedaily.com/releases/2013/02/130207131344.htm.

230   It helps stimulate white blood cells Hajo Haase and Lothar Rink, "The Immune System and the Impact of Zinc during Aging," *Immunity & Ageing* 6, no. 1 (2009), https://doi.org/10.1186/1742-4933-6-9.

230   the release and supply of neurotransmitters Lin Ren, Masoumeh Dowlatshahi Pour, Soodabeh Majdi, Xianchan Li, Per Malmberg, and Andrew G. Ewing, "Zinc Regulates Chemical-Transmitter Storage in Nanometer Vesicles and Exocytosis Dynamics as Measured by Amperometry," *Angewandte Chemie International Edition* 56, no. 18 (2017): 4970–75, https://doi.org/10.1002/anie.201700095.

230 according to one study on young adults Tamlin S. Conner, Aimee C. Richardson, and Jody C. Miller, "Optimal Serum Selenium Concentrations Are Associated with Lower Depressive Symptoms and Negative Mood among Young Adults," *Journal of Nutrition* 145, no. 1 (2014): 59–65, https://doi.org/10.3945/jn.114.198010.

230 needs selenium to function Gavin E. Arteel and Helmut Sies, "The Biochemistry of Selenium and the Glutathione System," *Environmental Toxicology and Pharmacology* 10, no. 4 (2001): 153–58, https://doi.org/10.1016/s1382-6689(01)00078-3.

230 Research has found a connection Jeremy W. Gawryluk, Jun-Feng Wang, Ana C. Andreazza, Li Shao, and L. Trevor Young, "Decreased Levels of Glutathione, the Major Brain Antioxidant, in Post-mortem Prefrontal Cortex from Patients with Psychiatric Disorders," *International Journal of Neuropsychopharmacology* 14, no. 1 (2010): 123–30, https://doi.org/10.1017/s1461145710000805.

230 Having ample levels of selenium Peter R. Hoffmann and Marla J. Berry, "The Influence of Selenium on Immune Responses," *Molecular Nutrition & Food Research* 52, no. 11 (2008): 1273–80, https://doi.org/10.1002/mnfr.200700330.

230 fermented foods support the production Ki-Bum Park and Suk-Heung Oh, "Production of Yogurt with Enhanced Levels of Gamma-Aminobutyric Acid and Valuable Nutrients Using Lactic Acid Bacteria and Germinated Soybean Extract," *Bioresource Technology* 98, no. 8 (2007): 1675–79, https://doi.org/10.1016/j.biortech.2006.06.006.

230 shown to change brain activity Kirsten Tillisch, Jennifer Labus, Lisa Kilpatrick, Zhiguo Jiang, Jean Stains, Bahar Ebrat, Denis Guyonnet, et al., "Consumption of Fermented Milk Product with Probiotic Modulates Brain Activity," *Gastroenterology* 144, no. 7 (2013), https://doi.org/10.1053/j.gastro.2013.02.043.

230 the same probiotics that nurture your gut Fang Yan and D. B. Polk, "Probiotics and Immune Health," *Current Opinion in Gastroenterology* 27, no. 6 (2011): 496–501, https://doi.org/10.1097/mog.0b013e32834baa4d.

230 people living with Alzheimer's "Probiotics Improve Cognition in Alzheimer's Patients," *Frontiers*, September 13, 2017, https://blog.frontiersin.org/2016/11/10/probiotics-improve-cognition-in-alzheimers-patients/.

230 Nourishes the gut microbiome Arthur C. Ouwehand, Seppo Salminen, and Erika Isolauri, "Probiotics: An Overview of Beneficial Effects," in *Lactic Acid Bacteria: Genetics, Metabolism and Applications*, eds. R. J. Siezen, J. Kok, T. Abee, and G. Schasfsma (SpringerLink: Springer, 2002), 279–89, https://doi.org/10.1007/978-94-017-2029-8_18.

231 Prebiotics help modulate the immune system F. Guarner, "Impacts of Prebiotics on the Immune System and Inflammation," *Diet, Immunity and Inflammation* (2013): 292–312. https://doi.org/10.1533/9780857095749.3.292.

231 They directly affect the immune cells E. N. Trushina, O. K. Mustafina, and D. B. Nikitiuk, "Limfoidnaia sistema kishechnika i immunomoduliruiushchee de-stvie prebio-tikov" [Intestinal lymphoid system and immunomodulating effects of prebiotics], *Voprosy pitaniia* 73, no. 6 (2004):49–53.

231 2019 research revealed Marcus Boehme, Marcel van de Wouw, Thomaz F. S. Bastiaanssen, Loreto Olavarría-Ramírez, Katriona Lyons, Fiona Fouhy, Anna V. Golubeva, et al., "Mid-life Microbiota Crises: Middle Age Is Associated with Pervasive Neuroimmune Alterations That Are Reversed by Targeting the Gut Microbiome, *Molecular Psychiatry* 25 (2020): 2567–83, https://doi.org/10.1038/s41380-019-0425-1.

231 Eating certain foods rich in melatonin Marie-Pierre St-Onge, Anja Mikic, and Cara Pietrolungo, "Effects of Diet on Sleep Quality," *Advances in Nutrition* 7, no. 5 (2016): 938–49, https://doi.org/10.3945/an.116.012336.

231 chill out without feeling groggy Christina Dietz and Matthijs Dekker, "Effect of Green Tea Phytochemicals on Mood and Cognition," *Current Pharmaceutical Design* 23, no. 19 (2017): 2876–2905, https://doi.org/10.2174/1381612823666170105151800.

231 boost your mood Natasha Gilbert, "The Science of Tea's Mood-Altering Magic," Outlook, *Nature*, February 6, 2019, https://www.nature.com/articles/d41586-019-00398-1

231 Dark chocolate contains some caffeine Andrew B. Scholey, Stephen J. French, Penelope J. Morris, David O. Kennedy, Anthea L. Milne, and Crystal F. Haskell, "Consumption of Cocoa Flavanols Results in Acute Improvements in Mood and Cognitive Performance during Sustained Mental Effort," *Journal of Psychopharmacology* 24, no. 10 (2009): 1505–14, https://doi.org/10.1177/0269881109106923.

231 caffeine can serve as what's known as a nootropic Joaquim A. Ribeiro and Ana M. Sebastião, "Caffeine and Adenosine," *Journal of Alzheimer's Disease* 20, no. s1 (2010), https://doi.org/10.3233/jad-2010-1379.

index

PATRICIA BANNAN, MS, RDN, is a nationally recognized registered dietitian nutritionist, healthy-cooking expert, and speaker. In addition to her nutrition credentials, she has conducted more than one thousand media interviews over the past decade, including guest appearances on the *Today* Show, *The Doctors,* and CNN. She resides in Los Angeles, California with her husband, children, and labradoodle, Pablo.